Jürgen Beyerer, Alexey Pak (Eds.)

Proceedings of the 2015 Joint Workshop of Fraunhofer IOSB and Institute for Anthropomatics, Vision and Fusion Laboratory

Karlsruher Schriften zur Anthropomatik
Band 24
Herausgeber: Prof. Dr.-Ing. Jürgen Beyerer

Lehrstuhl für Interaktive Echtzeitsysteme
Karlsruher Institut für Technologie

Fraunhofer-Institut für Optronik, Systemtechnik und
Bildauswertung IOSB Karlsruhe

Eine Übersicht aller bisher in dieser Schriftenreihe
erschienenen Bände finden Sie am Ende des Buchs.

Proceedings of the 2015 Joint Workshop of Fraunhofer IOSB and Institute for Anthropomatics, Vision and Fusion Laboratory

Edited by
Jürgen Beyerer
Alexey Pak

KIT Scientific Publishing

Impressum

KIT Scientific Publishing

Karlsruher Institut für Technologie (KIT)
KIT Scientific Publishing
Straße am Forum 2
D-76131 Karlsruhe

KIT Scientific Publishing is a registered trademark of Karlsruhe Institute of Technology. Reprint using the book cover is not allowed.

www.ksp.kit.edu

Print on Demand 2016

ISSN 1863-6489
ISBN 978-3-7315-0519-8
DOI 10.5445/KSP/1000054312

Preface

In 2015, the annual joint workshop of the Fraunhofer Institute of Optronics, System Technologies and Image Exploitation (IOSB) and the Vision and Fusion Laboratory (IES) of the Institute for Anthropomatics, Karlsruhe Institute of Technology (KIT) has again been hosted by the town of Triberg-Nussbach in Germany.

For a week from July, 19 to 26 the PhD students of the both institutions delivered extended reports on the status of their research and participated in thorough discussions on topics ranging from computer vision and world modeling to data fusion and human-machine interaction. Most results and ideas presented at the workshop are collected in this book in the form of detailed technical reports. This volume provides a comprehensive and up-to-date overview of the research program of the IES Laboratory and the Fraunhofer IOSB.

The editors thank Matthias Richter, Julius Pfrommer and other organizers for their efforts resulting in a pleasant and inspiring atmosphere throughout the week. We would also like to thank the doctoral students for writing and reviewing the technical reports as well as for responding to the comments and the suggestions of their colleagues.

Prof. Dr.-Ing. Jürgen Beyerer
Alexey Pak, PhD

Contents

Framework for Modeling Medical Guidelines Based on the Translation of UML Activities into YAWL

Patrick Philipp

Vision and Fusion Laboratory (IES)
Institute for Anthropomatics and Robotics (IAR)
Karlsruhe Institute of Technology (KIT), Germany
p.philipp@kit.edu

Technical Report IES-2015-01

Abstract: In several fields of the medical domain guidelines are used, opening up scope of actions for the medical practitioner. However, there is a gap between the theoretical knowledge they provide and practical solutions performed by the medical expert. Furthermore, barriers of implementation can arise. We propose a framework for modeling medical guidelines which takes these challenges into account. It is based on activities of the Unified Modeling Language (UML). These UML activities serve as an interface for more complex models, that can be used for advanced assistance functions. In this report we focus on translation rules transferring UML activities into Yet Another Workflow Language (YAWL).

1 Introduction

Guidelines are used in several fields of the medical domain – e.g. for the diagnosis of cancer [PFHB15a, PFHB15b, PFHB16]. Figure 1.1 depicts the stages of a medical guideline in such a context. Aside from the development and dissemination, the actual implementation of a guideline by the medical practitioner plays a decisive role.

That means, the medical expert has to adapt the recommendations to the given boundary conditions (patient, equipment, etc.)[FL92, SGM+11]. Consequently, there is a gap between the theoretical knowledge (provided by a guideline) on the one side and practical solutions (performed by the medical expert) on the other side. Additionally, barriers of guideline implementation can arise e.g. due to the fear of regimentation on part of the medical practitioner [PFHB15b].

Regardless of the specific medical domain, we propose a framework for modeling medical guidelines which allows the realization of assistance functions that reduce the gap between theoretical knowledge and practical solutions. To overcome barriers of guideline implementation, our modeling approach enables the medical expert to modify a guideline by him- or herself. Therefore, modifications – e.g. due to personal preferences or an individual surgical planning – can be incorporated in a guideline model.

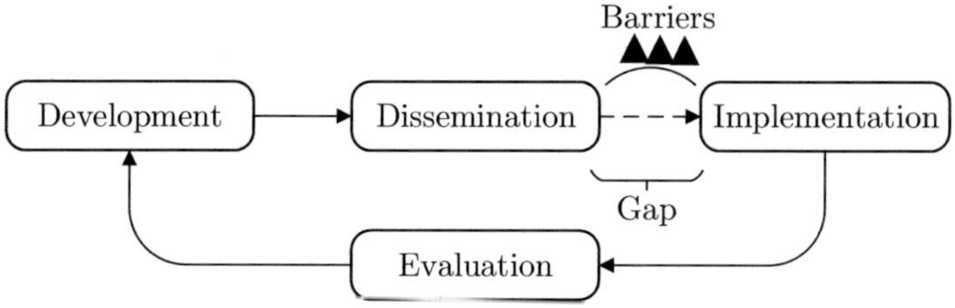

Figure 1.1: Stages of a medical guideline. The recommendations are developed and disseminated. However, there is a gap between theoretical knowledge and practical solutions carried out by the medical expert. Furthermore, barriers of guideline implementation can arise [PFHB16].

2 Modeling Approach

Typically, guidelines contain knowledge provided by schematic illustrations or continuous text that can not be translated into models offhand. We believe, that the formalization of this medical knowledge can be implemented by a dialog of experts (see Figure 2.1).

With the help of medical as well as technical domain experts, a guideline model in the form of an activity of the Unified Modeling Language (UML) is developed. A bypass is added to allow an interpretation of a guideline by the medical expert him- or herself. By proceeding in this way, barriers of guideline implementation are lowered.

In earlier publications ([PFHB15a, PFHB16]), we demonstrated the benefit of our approach by using only one comprehensible UML activity to (semi-) automatically generate more advanced models. These models, namely Petri nets and

Bayesian nets, where used to provide the actual assistance functions in context of a cancer diagnosis. These functions propose suitable examination values to the practitioner during the diagnostic process.

In our present work, we provide translation rules which transfer a UML activity of a medical guideline into a specification of Yet Another Workflow Language (YAWL). By this, a guideline can be used for assistance functions that are based on YAWL without the need to formalize it by using YAWL.

Despite the fact that intuitive YAWL editors for medical applications are developed [DHS$^+$16], we believe that our approach is more universal since it only relies on comprehensible UML activities for the process of formalization. This is the starting point to perform translation processes to elaborate more advanced models from just one given UML activity.

The automatic translation of a UML activity into a YAWL specification is based on the work of Han et. al [HZL10, HZLH12].

3 UML Activities

A huge benefit of UML is its acceptance in software industry worldwide [OMG11]. This, together with the fact that the syntax of UML activities is formalized and analyzed by various experts [RQ$^+$12] is one reason for choosing them as an interface in our framework. Furthermore, UML activities offer a high comprehensibility for the medical as well as the technical domain expert. This is a necessary precondition for making the experts' dialog work smoothly and to allow modifications by the medical expert on his own [PFHB15b].

3.1 Fundamentals

The 14 chart types which are offered by UML 2.4 can be divided into structural and behavioral diagrams [RQ$^+$12]. Activity diagrams are among the latter and therefore are able to answer the question of how a particular process or algorithm proceeds. To specify such an activity the modeler can use control flows, object flows, actions, decisions and forks [OMG11].

Typical routings appearing in the guideline models for cancer diagnosis are shown in [PFHB15a, PFHB15b, PFHB16]. With respect to the specification of general guideline models e.g. for surgical interventions, this common routings can be adopted. That is because the underlying principles of decision as well as sequential and parallel processing are the same. For an example refer to [BSRW16, SPG+16], where routings of surgical inventions for cholecystectomy (the removal of the gallbladder) or hip replacement are shown.

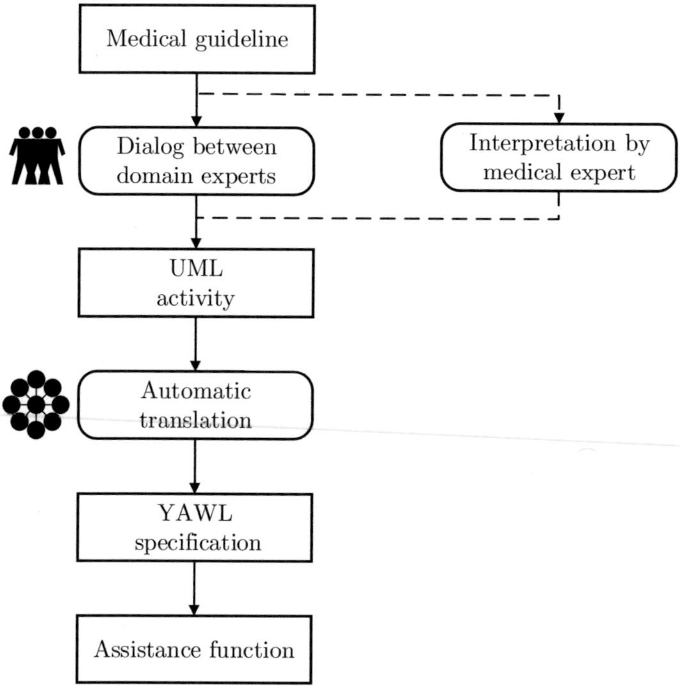

Figure 2.1: A medical guideline can be formalized via a dialog of experts from the medical as well as the technical domain. Additionally, the guideline can be interpreted by the medical expert on his- or her own.

Figure 3.1 depicts three typical routings appearing in the guideline models of cancer diagnosis shown in [PFHB15a, PFHB15b, PFHB16]. The initial node (black dot) represents the start of an activity whereas the activity final is represented by a double circle. Performed actions are shown as rounded rectangles, while the flow is represented by arrows.

Subfigure a) shows a case where actions are carried out sequentially (i.e. one after another). Subfigure b) depicts a selective routing. That means only one of the two actions A and B is performed. The corresponding decision is represented by a diamond (decision node) and depends in this example on a variable x which is either greater 1 or not. The second diamond is called a merge node as it merges the two possible flows.

Subfigure c) shows a routing where two actions can be performed concurrently. The flow is split up by a so called fork node (black bar on the left), whereas the join node (black bar on the right) synchronizes the two flows. The flow continues and therefore the activity ends, only if both actions have been performed in any arbitrary order [PFHB15b].

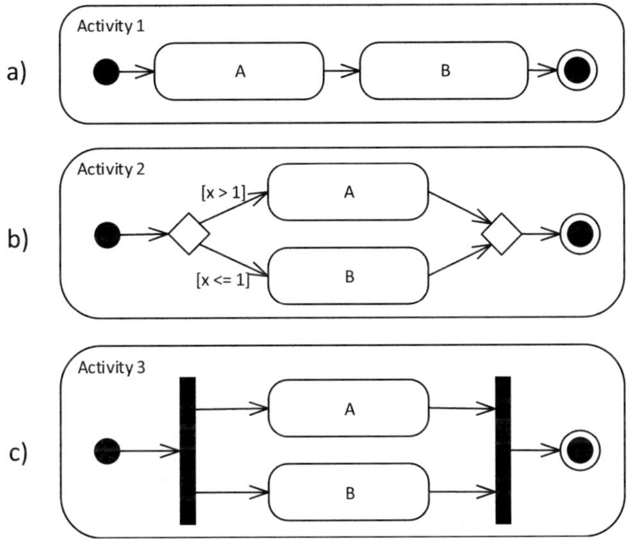

Figure 3.1: The three typical routings appearing in the guideline models of cancer diagnosis [PFHB16]. In Subfigure a) the actions A and B are performed sequentially (i.e. one after another). In Subfigure b) a decision has to be made in order to perform either A or B. Subfigure c) shows a routing where the actions A and B are performed concurrently. Consequently both actions are performed, but in any arbitrary order.

3.2 Modeling of Guidelines

Figure 3.2 depicts the model of a surgical intervention. More precisely, it is the model of a minimally invasive surgery: a cholecystectomy.

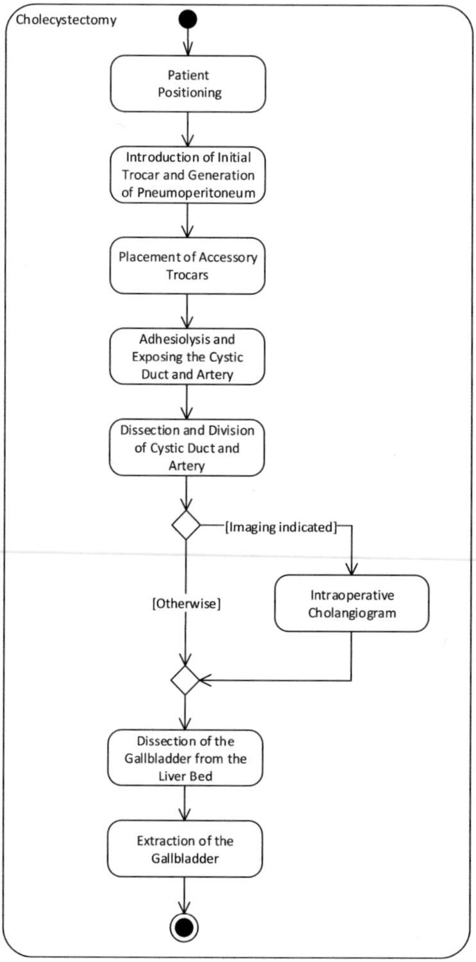

Figure 3.2: The UML activity of a cholecystectomy. At the biginning there is a sequential order of actions. The action "Intraoperative Cholangiogram" is optionally performed. The activity is derived from a graphical description in ref. [BSRW16].

In the upper part of this UML activity, a sequence of actions is shown (cf. subfigure a) in figure 3.1). Specifically, that means that the patient is positioned on the operating table. Then a sharpened tube to break through the abdominal wall

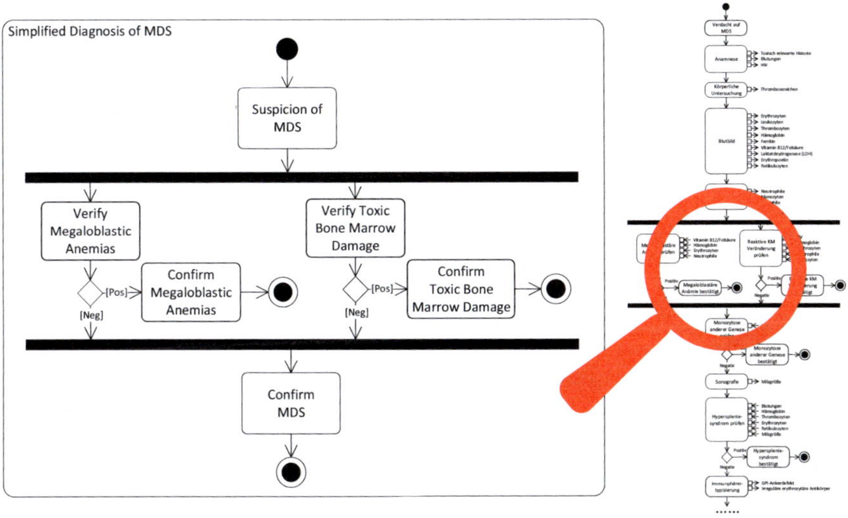

Figure 3.3: In the background of this figure, the first part of the diagnosis algorithm for blood cancer is shown [PFHB15b]. Because of the size of the guideline, a magnifying glass is used to emphasize the most important part – which is modeled as a stand-alone pseudo activity "Simplified Diagnosis of MDS". This activity will be used for the further translation process.

for the placement of other medical instruments (trocar) is used. By this, carbonic acid gas can be injected to inflate the abdomen.

After this, in action 3, more trocars are placed to enable the insertion of various medical instruments. In the following action, the cystic duct and the artery are exposed and clipped. As a consequence, they can be dissected in the subsequent action.

A decision has to be made, whether or not a radiographic imaging of the bile ducts with contrast medium (intraoperative cholangiogram) is performed (cf. subfigure b) in figure 3.1). After merging the two possible flows, another sequence of actions is performed, which includes the final extraction of the gallbladder.

Figure 3.3 shows a part of a diagnostic algorithm elaborated in [PFHB15b]. The corresponding activity basically consists of several sequences of actions and decisions. But in contrast to figure 3.2, there is a concurrent routing.

Moreover, there are several activity final nodes, i.e. the whole activity ends, if only one of the final nodes is executed. Since there are various final nodes inside the concurrent routing, all other (concurrent) actions are canceled as soon as the activity ends. For example, the depicted cutout in figure 3.3 shows two diagnoses: Megaloblastic Anemias and Toxic Bone Marrow Damage. Both of them can be excluded concurrently. Once one of these diagnoses is verified, the whole diagnostic algorithm ends. However, if none of these two diagnoses is verified, the diagnostic algorithm continues.

In the context of a surgical intervention such constructs can be used for an opt-out option, e.g. if some condition holds, the whole intervention is canceled.

4 YAWL

There are many reasons for choosing YAWL (Yet Another Workflow Language) as a target language for our framework [HRAA10]. One aspect is the expressive power and its formal semantics. Therefore analysis tools like WofYAWL [VvdAtH06] can be applied to verify the resulting model.

A key aspect is the use of YAWL as an intermediate language. I.e. the translated model can be used as an input for further assistance functions which are build upon a YAWL specification.

4.1 Fundamentals

A YAWL specification is a non-empty set of extended workflow nets (EWF-nets). An EWF-net is given by the following tuple [VvdAtH06, HRAA10]:

$$EWF = (i, o, C, T, F, f_{\text{split}}, f_{\text{join}}, f_{\text{rem}}, f_{\text{nofi}}) \,,$$

where

- $i \in C$ is the input condition,
- $o \in C$ is the output condition,
- C is a set of conditions,
- T is a set of tasks,
- $F \subseteq ((C \setminus \{o\}) \times T) \cup (T \times (C \setminus \{i\})) \cup (T \times T)$ is the flow relation,

- Every node in the graph $(C \cup T, F)$ is on a directed path from i to o,
- $f_{\text{split}} : T \rightsquigarrow \{\text{AND, OR, XOR}\}$ [1] specifies the split behavior of each task,
- $f_{\text{join}} : T \rightsquigarrow \{\text{AND, OR, XOR}\}$ specifies the join behavior of each task,
- $f_{\text{rem}} : T \rightsquigarrow \mathbb{P}^{+}(T \cup C \setminus \{i, o\})$ [2] specifies the tokens to be removed by emptying a part of the net,
- $f_{\text{nofi}} : T \rightsquigarrow \mathbb{N} \times \mathbb{N}^{\text{inf}} \times \mathbb{N}^{\text{inf}} \times \{\text{dynamic, static}\}$ specifies the multiplicity of each task.

4.2 Translation from UML Activity to YAWL

Given a UML activity represented as a graph $\mathcal{U} = (N, E)$. The set N can be further divided into different sets of nodes:

- $\mathcal{A}$: Set of actions,
- $\mathcal{I}, \mathcal{E}$: Set of initial node, set of final nodes,
- $\mathcal{B}$: Set of decision and merge nodes (branch nodes),
- $\mathcal{C}$: Set of fork and join nodes (concurrency nodes),
- $\mathcal{O}$: Set of object nodes.

The set of object nodes is given by the set of data pins. A node that is part of one of the node sets $\mathcal{S}, \mathcal{E}, \mathcal{B}, \mathcal{C}$ is called a control node. Furthermore, the set E is given by:

- $\mathcal{KF}$: Control flow, i.e. activity edges connecting actions and control nodes, as well as edges between themselves.
- $\mathcal{DF}$: Object flow, i.e. activity edges connecting actions and object nodes or between control nodes and object nodes.

[1] Please note: $\rightsquigarrow$ denotes a partial function. This means that a task can have no split behavior.

[2] Please note: $\mathbb{P}^{+}(X)$ denotes the power set of X without the empty set, i.e. $\mathbb{P}^{+}(X) = \mathbb{P}(X) \setminus \{\emptyset\}$

Formally the translation $[[\mathcal{U}]]$ of a UML activity $\mathcal{U}$ to an EWF-net is given by:

$$[[(N, E)]] = (i, o, C, T, F, f_{\text{split}}, f_{\text{join}}, f_{\text{rem}}, f_{\text{nofi}}),$$

where the graph $(C \cup T, F)$ is given by:

$$\begin{aligned}
i &= \mathcal{I}, && (4.1)\\
o &= c_{\text{out}}, && (4.2)\\
C &= \{i\} \cup \{o\}, && (4.3)\\
T &= \mathcal{A} \cup \{t_{\text{cncl}}\} \cup \{t_e \mid (e_1, e_2) \in \mathcal{KF}, \{e_1, e_2\} \cap \{\mathcal{B}, \mathcal{C}\} \neq \emptyset\}, && (4.4)\\
F &= \{\, (e_1, e_2) \mid (e_1, e_2) \in \mathcal{KF}, e_2 \notin \mathcal{E}, \\
&\qquad (e_1, e_2) \subseteq (\{o\} \times T) \cup (T \times \{i\}) \cup (T \times T) \,\} && (4.5)\\
&\quad \cup \{\, (e.\text{source}, t_e), (t_e, e.\text{target}) \mid e \in \mathcal{KF} \,\} && (4.6)\\
&\quad \cup \{\, (e_1, t_{\text{cncl}}) \mid (e_1, e_2) \in \mathcal{KF}, e_2 \in \mathcal{E} \,\} && (4.7)\\
&\quad \cup \{\, (t_{\text{cncl}}, c_{\text{out}}) \,\}. && (4.8)
\end{aligned}$$

Equation (4.1) shows, that the initial node $\mathcal{I}$ of a UML activity is translated into an input condition i of the EWF-net. This makes sense, since we assume that the corresponding UML activity has only one single initial node – just like the EWF-net has only one single input condition. Activity final nodes are not translated, instead one single output condition c_{out} is generated (4.2). That is, because we will bundle up all activity finals $\mathcal{F}$ in only one single condition (i.e. the output condition c_{out}). Finally, equation (4.3) shows, that the set of conditions C only consists of the input and the output condition since we do not need additional conditions for the translation process.

The set of tasks T results from the fact, that actions of the UML activity are translated into tasks of the EWF-net (4.4). Furthermore, an additional task t_{cncl} is added. This task is used to merge different flows of several activity finals of the corresponding UML activity. In addition, auxiliary tasks t_e are added to translate concurrency and branching nodes of the activity. These tasks are indexed by the edge e of the UML activity. This procedure is necessary, to be able to derive the flow relation in a further step.

The flow relation F contains all directed edges starting in e_1 and ending in e_2 – on the condition, that the edge is part of the activities' control flow and does not end in an activity final node (4.5). Moreover, the resulting edge must be valid in the sense that it is part of the flow specification. That means, for example, that there is no directed edge with the input condition as destination node (4.5).

All auxiliary tasks t_e are connected to their adjacent nodes by using the index e – i.e. for each task two edges are added (4.6). There is an edge $(e.\text{source}, t_e)$ having task t_e as target and there is another edge $(t_e, e.\text{target})$ having task t_e as source.

All directed edges of the UML activity pointing to a final node (at the same time the edge must be part of the control flow) are bend to one cancel task t_{cncl} of the resulting EWF-net (4.7). The cancel task t_{cncl} is connected to the output condition c_{out} (4.8).

After specifying the translation rules of the graph by equations (4.1) – (4.8), now, the functions $f_{\text{split}}, f_{\text{join}}, f_{\text{rem}}, f_{\text{nofi}}$ are defined. We are using the fact that a partial function $f' : X \rightsquigarrow Y$ with domain $\text{Dom}(f') \subseteq X$ can be modeled by a total function $f \colon X \to Y \cup \{\perp\}$ with domain $\text{Dom}(f) = X$:

$$f(x) = \begin{cases} f'(x), & \text{if } x \in \text{Dom}(f') \\ \perp, & \text{otherwise} \end{cases}$$

That means, we are using a total function f to model the partial behavior, i.e. only a subset $\text{Dom}(f')$ is mapped to an element of Y, whereas all other elements of $X \notin \text{Dom}(f')$ are mapped to $\perp$ (undefined). In our case, that means, we can define the necessary functions for all tasks $t \in T$:

$$f_{\text{split}}(t) = \begin{cases} \text{AND}, & \text{if } t = t_e : e = (e_1, e_2) \in \mathcal{KF}, e_2 \in \mathcal{C} \\ \text{XOR}, & \text{if } t = t_e : e = (e_1, e_2) \in \mathcal{KF}, e_2 \in \mathcal{B} \\ \perp, & \text{otherwise} \end{cases}$$

$$f_{\text{join}}(t) = \begin{cases} \text{AND}, & \text{if } t = t_e : e = (e_1, e_2) \in \mathcal{KF}, e_1 \in \mathcal{C} \\ \text{XOR}, & \text{if } t = t_{cncl} \vee t = t_e : e = (e_1, e_2) \in \mathcal{KF}, e_1 \in \mathcal{B} \\ \perp, & \text{otherwise} \end{cases}$$

$$f_{\text{rem}}(t) = \begin{cases} T \setminus \{t_{cncl}\}, & \text{if } t = t_{cncl} \text{ with } T \setminus \{t_{cncl}\} \neq \emptyset \\ \perp, & \text{otherwise} \end{cases}$$

$$f_{\text{nofi}}(t) = \perp$$

The function $f_{\text{split}}(t)$ specifies the split behavior of each task t. For newly added tasks t_e an AND split behavior is assigned, if the target e_2 of the edge e of the UML activity is a concurrency node. Additionally, an exclusive or (XOR) behavior is assigned if the target of edge e is a branch node. If a task t has no split behavior, it is assigned to $\perp$.

Analogously, the function $f_{\text{join}}(t)$ assigns an AND behavior if the source of an indexed task t_e is a concurrency node. And, if the source is a branch node, an XOR behavior is assigned. Finally, $\perp$ is assigned if task t has no join behavior.

The function $f_{\text{rem}}(t)$ assigns no removal behavior to all tasks t, except for task t_{cncl}. For this, it must hold: $T \setminus \{t_{\text{cncl}}\} \neq \emptyset$. I.e. no removal behavior is needed if no task t is present – consequently $f_{\text{rem}}(t)$ does not assign the empty set $\emptyset$. The removal behavior is needed, since all actions must be canceled as soon as an activity final is reached (cf. figure 3.3, page 7). Consequently, all tasks in the corresponding EWF-net must be canceled if task t_{cncl} is reached. Besides, since no task has a multiplicity, function $f_{\text{nofi}}(t)$ assigns all tasks t to $\perp$.

5 Verification

Figure 5.1 depicts the result of the translation rules applied to the UML guideline model of a cholecystectomy (cf. figure 3.2, page 6). The EWF-net starts with an input condition and ends with an output condition. The sequential order of actions has been directly translated into a sequential order of YAWL tasks.

One auxiliary task is added to model the decision node – another auxiliary task is added to model the merge node of the UML activity. In the first case the task is assigned to an XOR split behavior – in the latter case, an XOR join behavior is assigned. Figure 5.2 shows the result of the translation process for a simplified model of the diagnostic algorithm. As the UML activity ends if one activity final is executed, the corresponding YAWL model must comprise a cancellation area (dotted area) assigned to t_{cncl}. By this, all tasks inside the area can be canceled as soon as t_{cncl} is reached. That means, e.g., if "Toxic Bone Marrow Damage" is confirmed, all other tasks are canceled.

To sum up, we can say that the translation rules work as expected. Please note that figure 5.2 only depicts a simplified version of the diagnostic algorithm. Moreover, the UML data flow is omitted. Modeling the data flow is part of our future work – just like the extension of the YAWL model in figure 5.1 concerning probabilistic transitions to enable a situation detection based on various sensor data.

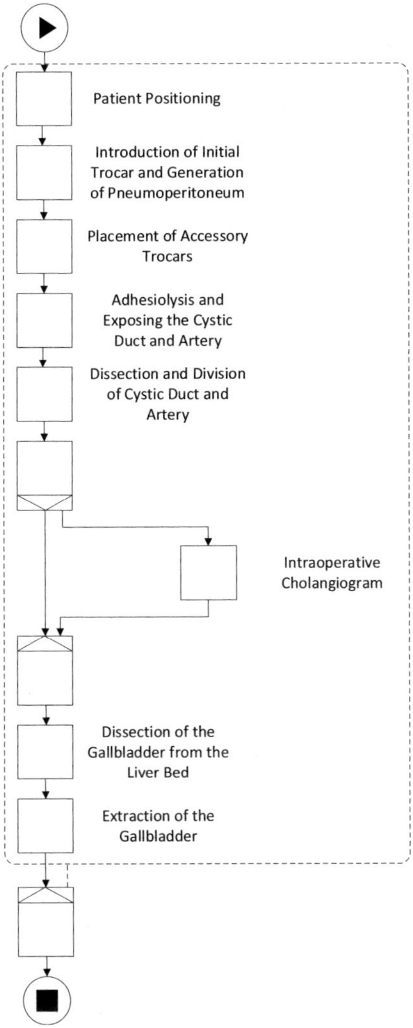

Figure 5.1: The model of a cholecystectomy after applying translation rules which transfer a UML activity to a YAWL specification. A sequential order of actions is translated into a sequential order of tasks. Auxiliary nodes are added to model a decision or a merge node.

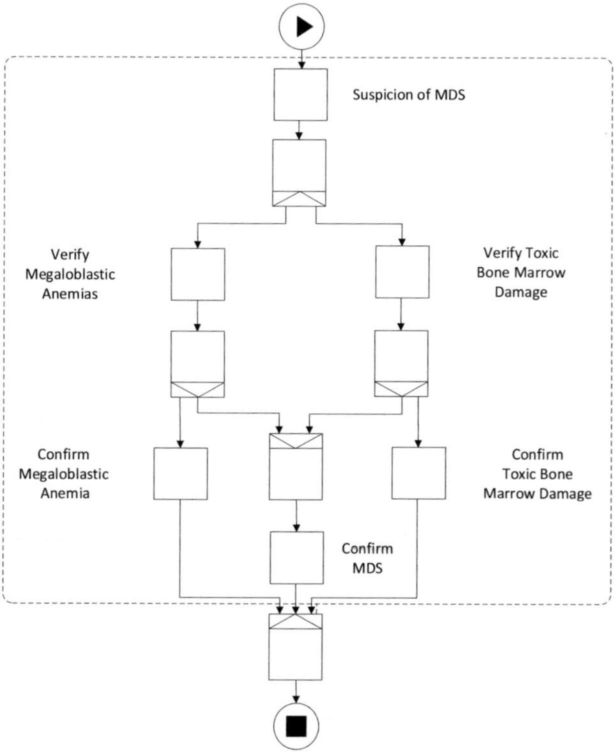

Figure 5.2: The simplified model of MDS diagnsosis after applying the proposed translation rules. Auxiliary nodes are added to model decision, fork and join nodes. Several edges are pointing to the cancel task, since the activity contains several final nodes.

6 Conclusion

In this technical report we introduced a framework for modeling medical guidelines. The framework utilizes UML activities as an interface for YAWL models. Activities are used because of their comprehensibility for the medical as well as the technical domain expert. By using only one comprehensible activity, several advanced models can be obtained by using translation rules. In the present work we focused on the translation of a UML activity into a YAWL specification. This specification can then be used as a basis for advanced assistance functions which are based on YAWL models.

Bibliography

[BSRW16] Andreas Bihlmaier, Luzie Schreiter, Jörg Raczkowsky, and Heinz Wörn. Hierarchical task networks as domain-specific language for planning surgical interventions. In *Intelligent Autonomous Systems 13*, volume 302 of *Advances in Intelligent Systems and Computing*, pages 1095–1105. Springer International Publishing, 2016.

[DHS+16] Simon Duerr, Anton Huck, Luzie Schreiter, Tim Beyl, Johannes Giehl, Markus Schwarz, Joerg Raczkowsky, and Heinz Woern. Intuitive workflow editor for owl based semantic networks in medical environment. *CARS*, 2016.

[FL92] E Field and K Lohr. *Guidelines for Clinical Practice: From Development to Use*. National Academies Press, Washington (DC), 1992.

[HRAA10] Arthur Hofstede, Nick Russell, Wil Aalst, and Michael Adams. *Modern Business Process Automation: YAWL and its Support Environment*. Springer, Berlin, 2010.

[HZL10] Zhaogang Han, Li Zhang, and Jiming Ling. Transformation of uml activity diagram to yawl. In *Enterprise Interoperability IV*, pages 289–299. Springer, Berlin, 2010.

[HZLH12] Zhaogang Han, Li Zhang, Jiming Ling, and Shihong Huang. Control-flow pattern based transformation from uml activity diagram to yawl. In *Enterprise Interoperability*, pages 129–145. Springer, Berlin, 2012.

[OMG11] OMG. OMG Unified Modeling Language(OMG UML) Superstructure Version 2.4.1, 2011.

[PFHB15a] Patrick Philipp, Yvonne Fischer, Dirk Hempel, and Jürgen Beyerer. Framework for an interactive assistance in diagnostic processes based on the translation of uml activities into petri nets. In *CSCI 2015, International Conference on Computational Science and Computational Intelligence: ISHI 2015, International Symposium on Health Informatics and Medical Systems, december 7-9*, pages 732–737. IEEE Conference Publishing Services, 2015.

[PFHB15b] Patrick Philipp, Yvonne Fischer, Dirk Hempel, and Jürgen Beyerer. Modeling of clinical practice guidelines for interactive assistance in diagnostic processes. In *WorldComp 2015, World Congress in Computer Science, Computer Engineering, and Applied Computing: HIMS 2015, International Conference on Health Informatics and Medical Systems, july 27-30*, pages 3–9. CSREA Press, 2015.

[PFHB16] Patrick Philipp, Yvonne Fischer, Dirk Hempel, and Jürgen Beyerer. *Emerging Trends in Computational Biology, Bioinformatics, and Systems Biology*, chapter Framework for an Interactive Assistance in Diagnostic Processes Based on Probabilistic Modeling of Clinical Practice Guidelines. Elsevier, 2016.

[RQ+12] Chris Rupp, Stefan Queins, et al. *UML 2 glasklar*. Carl Hanser Verlag GmbH Co KG, München, 2012.

[SGM+11] Earl Steinberg, Sheldon Greenfield, Michelle Mancher, et al. *Clinical Practice Guidelines We Can Trust*. National Academies Press, 2011.

[SPG+16] Luzie Schreiter, Patrick Philipp, Johannes Giehl, Yvonne Fischer, Markus Schwarz, Joerg Raczkowsky, Jürgen Beyerer, and Heinz Woern. Situation detection for an interactive assistance in surgical interventions based on random forests. *CARS*, 2016.

[VvdAtH06] HMW Verbeek, Wil MP van der Aalst, and Arthur HM ter Hofstede. Verifying workflows with cancellation regions and or-joins: an approach based on relaxed soundness and invariants. *The Computer Journal*, 50(3):294–314, 2006.

Linear Model for Optical Measurement

Ding Luo

Vision and Fusion Laboratory
Institute for Anthropomatics
Karlsruhe Institute of Technology (KIT), Germany
ding.luo@kit.edu

Technical Report IES-2015-02

Abstract: A linear measurement model is used to describe the measurement system where the measurements are linear combinations of the target signal. Due to its simplicity, it can be applied to various measurement systems. In this article, a comprehensive review of linear measurement model with a focus on optical systems is conducted by considering three different situations. Firstly, the assumption of signal sparsity is made, which turns the model into a compressive sensing problem. In spite of the various potentials demonstrated by the compressive sensing approach, it has been shown that compressive sensing is not fully ready for real-time applications yet due to its computational cost. Secondly, prior information of the target signal is taken into consideration to transform the linear measurement model into a linear manifold learning problem. With classical methods like principal component analysis (PCA), it has been demonstrated with two examples that such approach could simplify the measurement and the recovery process. Last but not least, the postprocessing step for the retrieval of information within the signal is further reduced through holistic design of the measurement system, granting systems with optical computation to make measurement faster and more robust against noise.

1 Introduction

Various real-world signals can be viewed as an n-dimensional vector $\mathbf{x} \in \mathbb{R}^n$, such as sound, image, etc. In a linear measurement model, each measurement of the target signal is a linear combination of all values in the vector $\mathbf{x}$. The complete measurements of the signal can be written as an m-dimensional vector $\mathbf{y} = A\mathbf{x} \in \mathbb{R}^m$ with an $m \times n$ measurement matrix A. Such formulation is very convenient as it covers many practical situations. For example, under the traditional Nyquist-Shannon sampling frame, the dimension of the signal $\mathbf{x}$ can be considered as tending to infinity, which represents a continuous function. Each row of the measurement matrix A is constructed as a bandpass filter which represents the sampling step.

The ultimate goal of the linear measurement model, like any other measurement systems, is to retrieve the signal $\mathbf{x}$ and the information it is carrying. Formulation of the linear measurement model as a linear system naturally leads to a classical problem of linear algebra: conditions for solving the equation $\mathbf{y} = A\mathbf{x}$. In this context, this problem is equivalent to determining which kind of measurements are needed in order to recover the signal.

According to the classical theory of linear algebra, if there are at least as many measurements as unknowns ($m \geq n$) and A has full rank, the problem is determined or overdetermined. Then the equation $\mathbf{y} = A\mathbf{x}$ can be solved uniquely (e.g. by Gaussian elimination). If there are fewer measurements than unknowns ($m < n$), the problem is underdetermined even with A having full rank. The knowledge of $\mathbf{y} = A\mathbf{x}$ restricts $\mathbf{x}$ to an affine subspace of $\mathbb{R}^n$, but does not determine $\mathbf{x}$ completely. Nevertheless, if A has full rank and $\mathbf{x}$ is believed to be "small", the least square approach yields $\mathbf{x}^{\#} = A^T(AA^T)^{-1}\mathbf{y}$, which is the solution of the ℓ_2-minimization problem:

$$\begin{aligned} \underset{\mathbf{z}}{\text{minimize}} \quad & \|\mathbf{z}\|_2 \\ \text{subject to} \quad & A\mathbf{z} = \mathbf{y} \end{aligned}$$

However, the assumption that the signal vector $\mathbf{x}$ is "small" does not apply to most of the signals in practice. Therefore, in order to solve an underdetermined linear system, many researchers have proposed various methods to solve this problem in unconventional ways, such as compressive sensing. This problem has profound practical value as the number of measurements could potentially be much smaller than the length of the signal to be measured.

The following content of the report is divided into several sections. In the second section, a theoretical review of compressive sensing is conducted with the help of an exemplary algorithm. The third section considers a more practical setting where prior information can be utilized to further simplify the recovery of the signal. In the fourth section, possibility is proposed that the information behind the signal can sometimes be retrieved directly without the recovery of the signal, which leads to a measurement system with optical computation capability.

2 Compressive Sensing

Compressive sensing (also known as compressed sensing, compressive sampling, or sparse sampling) consists of reconstructing an s-sparse vector $\mathbf{x} \in \mathbb{C}^N$ from $\mathbf{y} = A\mathbf{x}$, where $A \in \mathbb{C}^{m \times N}$ is the so-called measurement matrix representing an underdetermined linear system ($m < N$). Suppose vector $\mathbf{x}$ is the unique s-sparse solution of $A\mathbf{z} = \mathbf{y}$ with $\mathbf{y} = A\mathbf{x}$, the vector $\mathbf{x}$ can be reconstructed as the solution of:

$$\begin{aligned} &\underset{\mathbf{z} \in \mathbb{C}^N}{\text{minimize}} \quad \|\mathbf{z}\|_0 \\ &\text{subject to} \quad A\mathbf{z} = \mathbf{y} \end{aligned} \tag{2.1}$$

Unlike the assumption of the signal vector $\mathbf{x}$ as "small" mentioned in Sec. 1, the sparsity assumption is much more useful as it applies to most of the real-world signals. Many signals are naturally sparse, such as the signal from a heart beat monitor in the hospital where only values inside the peak are non-zero. For signals which are not sparse, there often exists a certain basis, with which the signal can be transformed into a sparse one. In the worst case, most of the signals can be well approximated by a sparse signal. This is the fundamental reason why compressive sensing has received increasing attention in recent years.

The problem of ℓ_0-minimization described by Eq. (2.1) can be split into two aspects. Firstly, it has to be guaranteed that the recovered signal $\mathbf{x}$ is the unique solution to the problem. Secondly, algorithms have to be developed to perform such recovery.

In order to fulfill the first condition, the measurement matrix has to be constructed according to the sparsity of the signal. This involves both the size of the signal, which is directly linked to the number of measurements, and the property of the matrix. Generally speaking, the measurement matrix has to be *incoherent*, in order to guarantee that the reconstruction is unique [FR13]. The Restricted Isometry Property (RIP) proposed by Emmanuel J. Candes [Can08] is generally considered as a canonical measure of the coherence of a measurement matrix. Deliberate construction of a matrix with RIP is a very hard problem but fortunately with statistical tools it has been proven that random matrices tend to have RIP with high probability [FR13].

The progress of algorithm development for ℓ_0-minimization problem has not been easy as it has been proven that the problem is NP-hard [FR13]. The breakthrough is made by Emmanuel J. Candes *et al.* with their discovery of theoretically guaranteed equivalence between ℓ^0-minimization and ℓ^1-minimization under certain conditions [CRT06]. This leads to a branch of optimization methods based on ℓ^1-minimization, often referred to as Basis Pursuit. As a convex optimization problem, it can be solved fairly fast with linear programming methods. Another major branch of methods are greedy methods, based on iterative construction/modification/thresholding of the support of $\mathbf{x}$, such as Orthogonal Matching Pursuit [TG07] and Iterative Hard Thresholding [BD09].

As a fairly new paradigm, compressive sensing has shown great potential. Firstly, the linear sampling scheme serves as an alternative to the traditional Nyquist-Shannon sampling theory, which allows for much reduced number of measurements under many situations. Secondly, the optimization nature of compressive sensing grants itself intrinsic tolerance against noise, which is very important in practical situations. Such features have helped to realize the application of compressive sensing in various fields, especially in optical imaging/measurement led by the development of the single-pixel camera [DDT+08].

In spite of its popularity, there are various factors preventing compressive sensing from being applied in real-time measurement systems. To begin with, the computational cost of the reconstruction algorithms is still relatively high, in terms of both time and space. Since most algorithms are based on iterative processes in an optimization loop and each step often consists of considerable amount of computational task, the reconstruction process is very time consuming even for state-of-the-art algorithms, which are already thousands of times faster than primary algorithms invented at the beginning of compressive sensing. For example, TVAL3 is an algorithm developed by Chengbo Li with the specific target of image reconstruction [Li09], which can be applied in implementations like single pixel camera. Although it is among the fastest and best performing algorithms for compressive sensing, reconstruction of a single image with 64×64 pixels using 30% measurements still takes 1.9 second on a consumer laptop. To increase the size of the image to 640×640 pixels, the measurement matrix would be 122880×409600 large and takes a memory space of 375GB with double precision. Additionally, empirical experiences have shown that the efficiency of the algorithms relies heavily on the tuning of the input parameters. Therefore, it is in the author's opinion that compressive sensing is still not ready for real-time measurement areas.

3 Linear Manifold Learning

Conventional compressive sensing theories rely only on the sparsity of the signal, whereas in reality more a priori information could be linked to the target signal to facilitate reconstruction. To further utilize such information, model-based compressive sensing is proposed by R.G. Baraniuk *et al.* [BCDH10], where dependencies between values and locations in the signal are taken into consideration to allow for even less measurements with robust recovery.

To push it even further, in the extreme case that all possible forms of the signal are known a priori, the linear measurement model can be transformed into a linear manifold learning problem, denoted by $Y = AX$, where $X \in \mathbb{R}^{n \times p}$ contains p possible n-dimensional signals and $Y \in \mathbb{R}^{m \times p}$ contains p corresponding m-dimensional measurements, which are linked through the linear measurement matrix $A \in \mathbb{R}^{m \times n}$. Since X is considered known a priori, various linear methods can be used to construct the measurement matrix A to yield best measurements for recovery, such as principal components analysis, metric multidimensional scaling, etc.

3.1 Chromatic Confocal Signal

In a chromatic confocal system, an objective lens with controlled chromatic aberration is used to separate different spectral components of the illumination light on to different focal planes. The reflected light from the sample, after the confocal filtering, will be concentrated around the spectral component that is in focus, generating a quasi-Gaussian peak in the spectrum, which is traditionally measured with a spectrometer.

In a predefined optical system, such quasi-Gaussian peaks can be considered as known a priori. All possible peak functions can be collected to form the matrix X. Principal component analysis can be performed on matrix X yielding a series of principal components, the largest of which are used to construct the measurement matrix A. The pseudo-inverse matrix of A can be applied on the measurement Y for the reconstruction of the signals: $X_R = A^T Y = A^T AX$.

As shown by the simulation results in Fig. 3.1, it is possible to recover the shape of the peak function with only three linear measurements. Due to the fact that the calculation of the pseudo-inverse of A is rank deficient, $A^T A$ is not an identity matrix, thus the reconstruction is not exact. Nevertheless, the peak position is well aligned with the original signal, and therefore preserving the information within. By increasing the number of linear measurements, the recovery accuracy will be much improved.

With application of the linear measurement model on a chromatic confocal setup, the spectrometer with thousands of pixels could potentially be replaced by a limited set of filter combinations, allowing much less data flow and thus increased measurement speed. Compared with conventional compressive sensing, the reconstruction process is dramatically simplified as it involves only matrix multiplication.

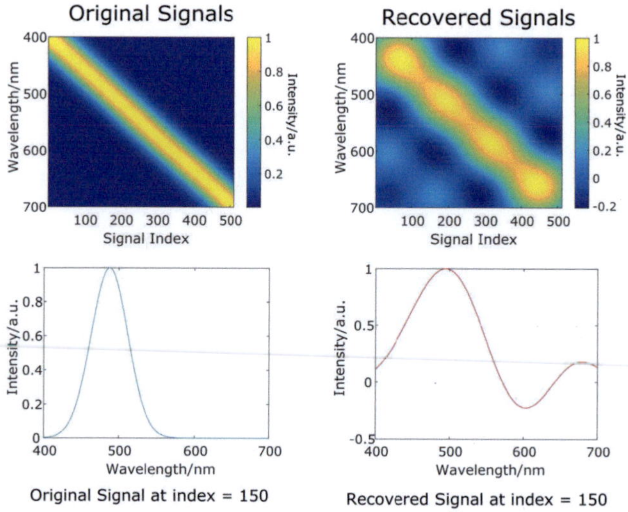

Figure 3.1: Simulation results of Gaussian signals.

3.2 Shape from Focus

Shape from focus is yet another field where linear measurement model with prior information could potentially be applied to enhance the efficiency of the technique. Depending on the size of the aperture, focal length of the objective, focal plane position and size of the imaging pixel, an imaging system has a certain depth of focus so that objects out of focus get blurred. The measure of how well an object is in focus can serve as a datum for measuring the distance of this object to the imaging system. When the measurement is taken across the complete field of the imaging system, the three dimensional profile of the object surface could be retrieved.

Conventional shape from focus methods generally involve several steps. Firstly, an image sequence is captured while the focal plane of the imaging system is shifted by either mechanical scanning of camera/sample or motorized focus shifting within the objective lens. Secondly, focus measure values for each pixel in every image are computed to construct a 3D data cube with 2D transverse spatial coordinates corresponding to camera pixels and 1D axial shift coordinate. Various algorithms have been developed for this purpose [PPG13]. Lastly, the 3D profile of the sample is reconstructed from these focus measure values in the data cube. This can be conducted through either simple approaches like taking axial location with maximum focus value as the target position [PPG13], or with more sophisticated approaches by encoupling optimization algorithms such as Total Variation regularization [Mah13].

Regardless of the focus measure algorithms, the focus measure values of one specific pixel at different axial locations typically form a quasi-Gaussian shape, similar to that of the (chromatic) confocal signal. Therefore in principal, it is possible to apply the same linear measurement model to the process of shape from focus. Instead of taking a complete sequence of axially shifted images, only a limited number of images are required, which are linear combinations of the original image sequence. The complete focus measure signal can be retrieved from the focus measure of these synthetic images provided that the focus measure operation is linear.

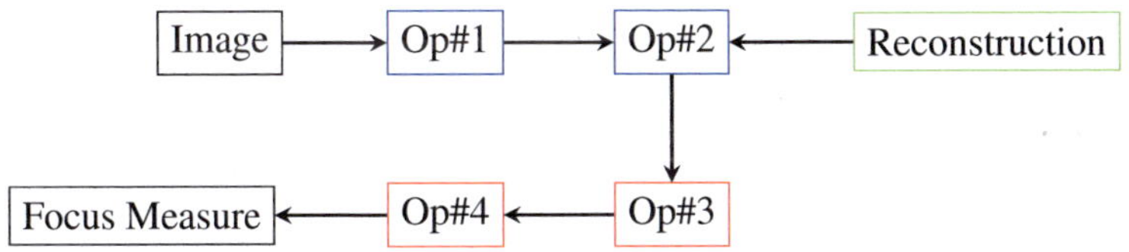

Figure 3.2: Exemplary processes of shape from focus with linear measurement model. Op#1 and Op#2 are linear operations on the image while Op#3 and Op#4 are non-linear.

However, modern focus measure algorithms often consist of multiple steps of operations on the image, many of which are non-linear operations. This prevents direct recovery of the original focus measure signal from the synthetic images. Nevertheless, for an algorithm with multiple steps of operations, as long as there exists one linear operation before all non-linear steps, a reconstruction step can be inserted to recover not the focus measure value directly, but rather the result of the last linear operation. An example is illustrated by the diagram in Fig. 3.2.

Fortunately, many efficient focus measure algorithms indeed have at least one linear operation before all non-linear operations. Take the Modified Laplacian (LAPM) for example [PPG13]. A one dimensional Laplacian filter $M = [-1\ 2\ -1]$ is firstly constructed. Then the image is filtered in both x and y directions respectively. The absolute value of the two filtered images are summed as the final focus measure value. Apparently the 1D filtering operation as a convolution is linear while taking the absolute value is non-linear. Therefore the reconstruction step must be inserted before taking the absolute value.

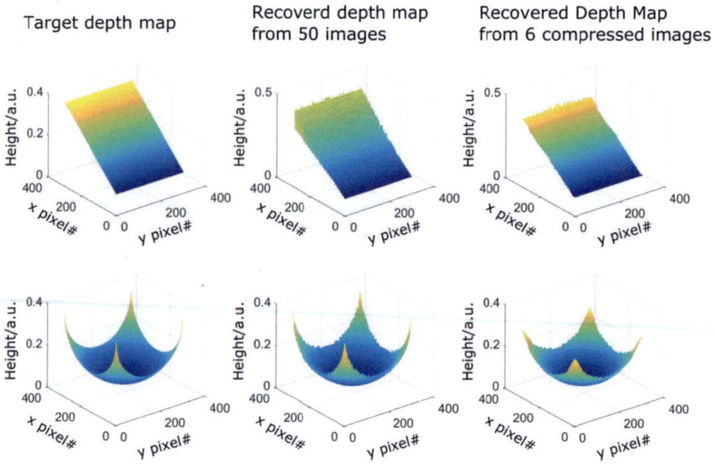

Figure 3.3: Simulation result of compressed shape from focus.

Simulation with this method is performed with synthetic images for two surface profiles. One is a linear ramp while the other one is part of a sphere. Both surface profiles are overlaid with the same texture map for the synthesizing of an axial image sequence with 50 images. With the conventional shape from focus method, LAPM is applied to all 50 images for focus measure, and axial position with the maximum value is taken as the axial position for each pixel. Meanwhile, based on the prior information provided by LAPM and the imaging system, a measurement matrix is constructed to linearly combine the image sequence to form six compressed images. LAPM is applied to these six images with reconstruction before the absolute value operation. The result of both approaches are illustrated in Fig. 3.3. It is clearly demonstrated that such compressed measurement yields comparable result to conventional methods, but largely reduces the number of images to be taken as well as the following image processing tasks.

In practice, the realization of the linear measurement can be achieved in many different ways. One possible implementation is to take a chromatic objective coupled with spectrally filtered illumination/detection. Another approach could be to change the focus position within each exposure with varying speed derived from the constructed measurement matrix, possibly through liquid lenses.

Fundamentally, the conventional compressive sensing is closely related to such linear measurement model with prior knowledge. Both can be compared in a classical linear algebra picture. Conventional compressive sensing considers the linear projection from *a collection of hyperplanes* (derived from *sparsity of the signal*) to a lower dimensional manifold and the recovery of the point in such *hyperplanes* through its counter part in such lower dimensional manifold. As a manifold learning problem, linear measurement model with prior knowledge considers the linear projection from *a particular subspace* (derived from *prior knowledge of the signal*) to a lower dimensional manifold and the recovery of the point in such *subspace* through its counter part in such lower dimensional manifold.

4 Optical Computation

It has been shown that with the linear measurement model, the process of conducting a measurement is much simplified. In compressive sensing, this is realized under the assumption of the signal sparsity while in a linear manifold learning problem, this is achieved with the help of prior knowledge. Nevertheless, signal reconstruction is a necessary step in both approaches.

Fig. 4.1 lists three different information embedding and recovery schemes. In the first case, the signal to be measured and the information to be retrieved are equivalent, for example an image taken for the pure target of recording the scene. In most situations, the information and the signal are not exactly the same thing, like illustrated in the second and third cases. Both Sec. 2 and Sec. 3 are dealing with the second case where the signal is reconstructed from the measurement and then a postprocessing step is implemented to retrieve the target information from the signal. This is often not the optimum case since the process between measurement and signal and the process between signal and information are treated separately. In this section, a different approach is proposed to treat the complete process holistically to further improve the efficiency of the measurement. A major assumption made beforehand is that in many practical measurement scenarios, the information embedded in the signal residing in a high dimensional manifold is often of lower dimensions by itself.

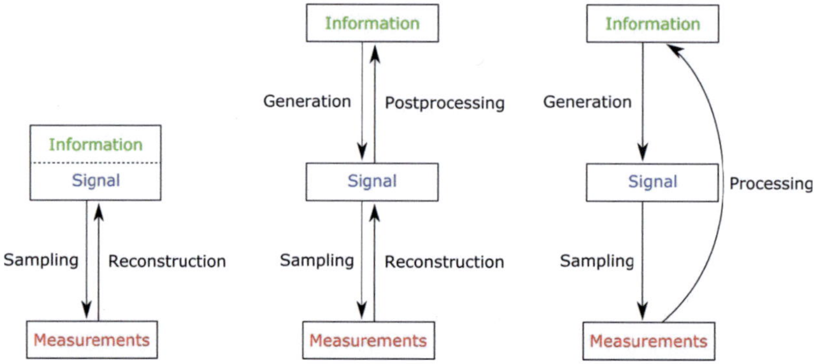

Figure 4.1: Different information embedding and recovery schemes.

Take the quasi-Gaussian signal for example. In the scenarios discussed in previous sections, a one dimensional target information, the axial position of the sample, is embedded in this peak function with a non-linear and implicit manner. After the peak function (signal) is reconstructed from the measurement, a further step is required to retrieve the information, such as through the location of the peak/centroid of the signal.

In fact, this postprocessing step can be effectively reduced/minimized by coupling it into the sampling process. To retrieve the centroid of the signal, a "centroid" preserving measurement matrix can be constructed for the measurement. Construction of such a matrix can be performed using Bernstein Polynomials.

For example, Fig. 4.2 illustrates the measurement results of a Gaussian signal with measurement matrices constructed from Bernstein Polynomials of different degrees. Regardless of the degrees of the polynomials, it can be proven mathematically that the measurement always preserves the centroid of the original signal. One idea to implement such a measurement is to build a chromatic probe using one linear interference filter as the first degree Bernstein polynomial. In this case the height of the sample can be retrieved with minimum processing. Schematic of such optical system is shown in Fig. 4.3

The fundamental difference of this approach with respect to the approaches proposed in previous sections is that the computation/processing part is largely shifted to the optical system through holistic design of the measurement setup.

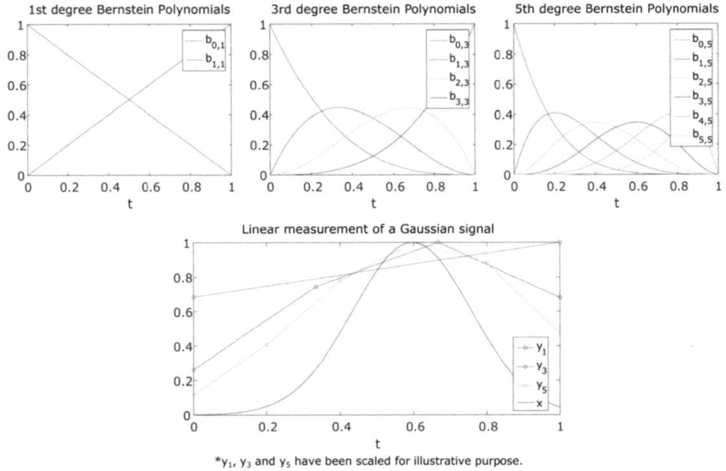

Figure 4.2: Linear measurement of a Gaussian signal with different degrees of Bernstein Polynomials.

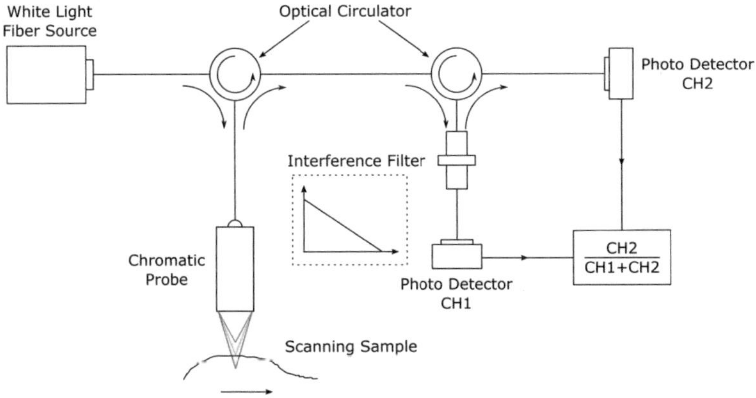

Figure 4.3: Schematic of a two-channel chromatic confocal measurement setup using first degree Bernstein Polynomials to retrieve centroid location directly.

In the proposed chromatic system, the measurement matrix is achieved by optical filters. This not only alleviates the computational burden in many systems, but more importantly, reduces the effect of the optoelectronic noises which propagates in the processing chain in conventional optical measurement systems.

5 Conclusion

The discussion presented in this paper is centered around the linear measurement model $\mathbf{y} = A\mathbf{x}$, where the measurements are linear combinations of the target signal. By making the assumption that the target signal is sparse, this model turns into a compressive sensing problem. In spite of the potential it has demonstrated, the computational cost has prevented compressive sensing from being applied in real-time measurement systems at the moment. With prior information of target signal taken into consideration, the linear measurement model is transformed into a linear manifold learning problem, where classical methods like PCA can be utilized to construct the measurement matrix which allows direct recovery of the signal from the measurement. Examples of chromatic confocal measurement and shape from focus are presented to demonstrate the potential of such approach in real world optical measurement systems. Last but not least, a holistic approach is proposed in order to retrieve the information with minimum postprocessing, allowing optical computation in measurement systems, which is both faster and more robust against noise.

Bibliography

[BCDH10] R.G. Baraniuk, V. Cevher, M.F. Duarte, and C. Hegde. Model-based compressive sensing. *Information Theory, IEEE Transactions on*, 56(4):1982–2001, 4 2010.

[BD09] Thomas Blumensath and Mike E. Davies. Iterative hard thresholding for compressed sensing. *Applied and Computational Harmonic Analysis*, 27(3):265 – 274, 2009.

[Can08] Emmanuel J. Candes. The restricted isometry property and its implications for compressed sensing. *Comptes Rendus Mathematique*, 346(9-10):589 – 592, 2008.

[CRT06] Emmanuel J. Candes, Justin K. Romberg, and Terence Tao. Stable signal recovery from incomplete and inaccurate measurements. *Communications on Pure and Applied Mathematics*, 59(8):1207–1223, 2006.

[DDT+08] M.F. Duarte, M.A. Davenport, D. Takhar, J.N. Laska, Ting Sun, K.F. Kelly, and R.G. Baraniuk. Single-pixel imaging via compressive sampling. *Signal Processing Magazine, IEEE*, 25(2):83–91, 3 2008.

[FR13] Simon Foucart and Holger Rauhut. *A mathematical introduction to compressive sensing*. Springer, 2013.

[Li09] Chengbo Li. *An efficient algorithm for total variation regularization with applications to the single pixel camera and compressive sensing*. PhD thesis, Rice University, 2009.

[Mah13] M.T. Mahmood. Shape from focus by total variation. In *IVMSP Workshop, 2013 IEEE 11th*, pages 1–4, 6 2013.

[PPG13] Said Pertuz, Domenec Puig, and Miguel Angel Garcia. Analysis of focus measure operators for shape-from-focus. *Pattern Recognition*, 46(5):1415 – 1432, 2013.

[TG07] J.A. Tropp and A.C. Gilbert. Signal recovery from random measurements via orthogonal matching pursuit. *Information Theory, IEEE Transactions on*, 53(12):4655–4666, 12 2007.

An Unsupervised Domain Adaptation Concept for Face Recognition Applications

Christian Herrmann

Vision and Fusion Laboratory
Institute for Anthropomatics
Karlsruhe Institute of Technology (KIT), Germany
christian.herrmann@kit.edu

Technical Report IES-2015-03

Abstract: When facing real world data, domain shift is a significant challenge for face recognition methods. A domain mismatch between the datasets used to train a recognition model in the lab and the target data leads to a negative impact on the performance of the recognitions system. Because it is difficult for some domains, like surveillance footage, to collect sufficiently large training datasets, a concept to generalize from data originating from a set of given domains to novel domains is proposed. The critical difference to most existing learning strategies under these conditions is the additional constraint that no data is available from the target domain which is called unsupervised domain adaptation. The suggested concept combines large-margin dimension reduction with an SVM-based framework for unsupervised domain adaptation. This unified strategy benefits by using more of the available knowledge about the training data in the sense of dataset/domain membership of the training samples compared to simply combining all available training datasets into one large dataset.

1 Introduction

When considering practical applications of face recognition systems, one faces a rather obvious, but tough problem. In contradiction to scientific evaluations, where training and testing is performed on the same dataset, *e.g.* the well-known Labeled Faces in the Wild (LFW) [HRBLM07] or YouTube Faces Database (YTF) [WHM11] benchmarks, systems that will eventually be shipped to a costumer need to generalize from a specific dataset, *i.e.* the training data must be generalized in a way that solving the trained task on novel data coming from a different domain is still possible. Current scientific and publicly available datasets were often collected from professional sources such as TV, movies, newspapers, magazines or commercials, because such data is easily accessible in large amounts through the Internet nowadays. This includes the image data as well as according meta data regarding the identity of the shown persons, basically eliminating the necessity for manual annotation of the data. On the other hand, there are the domains where face recognition should be applied, most prominently private smartphone shots or videos and surveillance data, where the collection of similar amounts of annotated data suitable for training purposes is very hard. This is mostly restricted by privacy and economical reasons. First, privacy issues preventing the easy collection of large amounts of such data and, second, due to the lack of meta data, the economic inefficiency to manually prepare the collected data with annotations for training purposes. This means, the inherent differences between the data from different domains are also existent between the training data and the application data of a face recognition system. There are obvious differences like a wider range of head poses in surveillance data compared to TV data, and less obvious ones like artistic color corrections in movies or failed white balancing in low-quality smartphone cameras.

This problem of domain shift is well-known [QCSSL09, PGLC15] and adaptation strategies under favorable conditions are quite popular and known as Semi-supervised Learning, Transfer Learning, Self-taught Learning or Covariate Shift, depending on how much and what specific information is available from the training domains and the target domain [PGLC15]. Semi-supervised Learning, for example, assumes fully annotated data from the training domains and unlabeled data from the target domain.

In the addressed case of face recognition, we are challenged by the tougher problem of unsupervised domain adaptation, where fully annotated data from the training domains is assumed, but no data at all from the target domain. This prevents the common strategy of learning a complete model from the training data and then adjusting the model to the target domain by re-training with data out of it. The problem of unsupervised domain adaptation can only be solved by proper generalization from the training data and that is where a lot of current supervised face recognition systems fail. In the case of object classification, the problem was prominently illustrated a few years ago [TE+11], however, the number of potential solutions remained limited [KZM+12, GLC11, FHST13]. In terms of face recognition, this issue appears to be out of the scientific focus.

To address this lack of attention, we present a modification of the unsupervised domain adaptation method proposed by [KZM+12] to match the scenario of face recognition. The method from [KZM+12] is an extension of a linear SVM and thus able to solve classification problems. Using the large-margin dimension reduction concept from [HB15a, SPVZ13] and combining it with the unsupervised domain adaptation makes this approach suitable for face recognition tasks. The main benefit of the proposed strategy compared to a combined learning on all available training datasets is the better usage of the available information. It specifically uses the information which domain (*i.e.* training dataset) each sample comes from, which can be seen as an additional label. So instead of only using the identity label for each training sample when doing a combined training, the domain adaptation training strategy uses the identity label as well as the domain label of each training sample to get a better generalization. Getting this domain label comes at no additional cost because the knowledge that samples from different datasets come from different domains is used. This results in better usage of the limited training data.

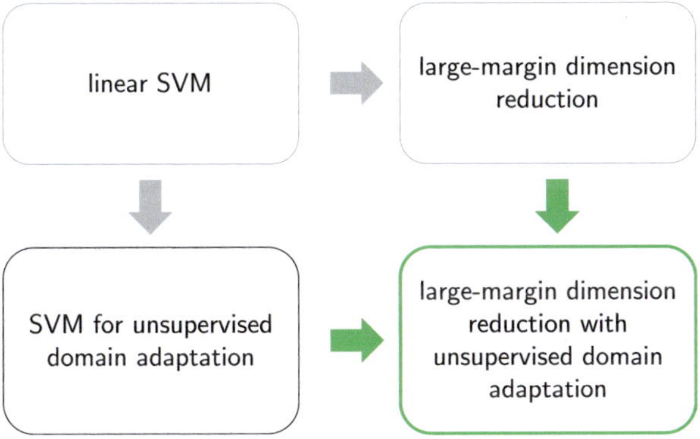

Figure 2.1: Both combined approaches are based on the linear SVM.

2 Unsupervised domain adaptation for face recognition

Previously, we published a face recognition system suitable for low-resolution and large scale data [HB15a]. The key component in terms of machine learning is a linear dimension reduction of high dimensional fisher vectors φ to low dimensional target vectors $\boldsymbol{v}$ by a matrix W: $\boldsymbol{v} = W\varphi$. The projection matrix W is trained by stochastic sub-gradient descent and a max-margin based loss function, which will be explained in detail later on. Consequently, this part has to be robust against domain shifts. The difficulty in terms of face recognition applications is usually that no data is available from the target domain, leading to the demand of an unsupervised domain adaptation approach. The concept proposed by [KZM+12] can be merged with the previously used dimension reduction strategy because they are both based on the linear SVM (Fig. 2.1). In the following sections the principle of the base methods are revisited in the necessary detail and finally combined into the proposed approach.

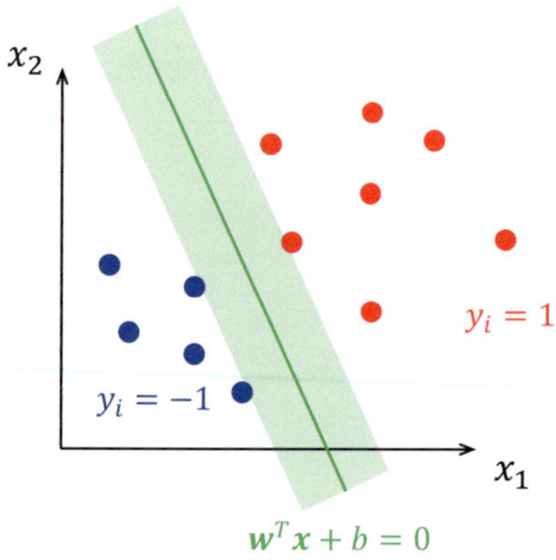

Figure 2.2: Basic concept of a linear SVM: maximizing the margin (bright green) around the hyperplane (green) to separate the feature vectors from two classes (red and blue).

2.1 Linear SVM

Given is a set of feature vectors $\{\boldsymbol{x}_1, \dots, \boldsymbol{x}_n\}$, each describing an object that belongs to one of two classes. Let $y_i = \{-1, 1\}$ be the indicator to which class the object that is described by $\boldsymbol{x}_i$ belongs. Then the basic idea of a linear SVM for classification is to find a separating hyperplane $\boldsymbol{w}^T \boldsymbol{x} + b = 0$ in the feature space that maximizes the margin between the samples of both classes as shown by Fig. 2.2. The maximization of the margin can be formulated as

$$\min_{\boldsymbol{w},b} \frac{1}{2} ||\boldsymbol{w}||_2^2 \quad , \text{ where } y_i \cdot \left(\boldsymbol{w}^T \boldsymbol{x}_i + b\right) \geq 1, \ \forall i. \tag{2.1}$$

This constrained optimization problem is hard to solve, which is why the hinge loss l is a popular choice for the loss function for the optimization:

$$l = \sum_i \max\left(0, 1 - y_i \cdot \left(\boldsymbol{w}^T \boldsymbol{x}_i + b\right)\right). \tag{2.2}$$

Loss minimization can then be performed by stochastic sub-gradient descent. The update step using the learning rate α is given by

$$\boldsymbol{w}_{t+1} = \begin{cases} \boldsymbol{w}_t & \text{, for } 1 - y_i \cdot \left(\boldsymbol{w}^T \boldsymbol{x}_i + b\right) < 0 \\ \boldsymbol{w}_t + \alpha y_i \boldsymbol{x}_i & \text{, otherwise} \end{cases}.$$

2.2 Unsupervised domain adaptation

Khosla et al. presented a strategy to extend the basic linear SVM to unsupervised domain adaptation [KZM+12]. Based on the typical scenario that only a limited amount of training datasets, each from a different domain D_k, is available, the authors construct a framework that tries to generalize from the set of these domain-specific datasets to data from novel domains. The basic assumption is that each domain D_k is only a part of the visual world V and each domain D_k has a bias vector $\boldsymbol{\Delta}_k$, common for all examples from that domain, that describes the bias of this domain compared to the visual world. A domain specific model $\boldsymbol{w}_k$ is built by the sum of the global visual world model $\boldsymbol{w}_g$ and the domain specific bias $\boldsymbol{\Delta}_k$. Under the assumption that the bias is captured in the feature space and the same feature space is used for all domains, the authors propose an SVM-based framework to address the domain bias. A set of $n+1$ SVMs is trained for n available training domains, including one local SVM for each domain and additionally one for the visual world. The local SVMs are modeled as

$$\boldsymbol{w}_k = \boldsymbol{w}_g + \boldsymbol{\Delta}_k \tag{2.3}$$

leading to a coupled formulation and training of all $n+1$ SVMs. The basic linear SVM equation (2.1) is extended to

$$\min_{\boldsymbol{w}_g, \boldsymbol{\Delta}_k, b_g, b_k} \frac{1}{2}||\boldsymbol{w}_g||_2^2 + \frac{\lambda}{2} \sum_{k=1}^{n} ||\boldsymbol{\Delta}_k||_2^2 \quad \text{, where} \tag{2.4}$$
$$y_i \cdot \left(\boldsymbol{w}_g^T \boldsymbol{x}_{ik} + b_g\right) \geq 1, \;\; i = 1, \ldots, s_k \text{ and } k = 1, \ldots, n$$
$$y_i \cdot \left(\boldsymbol{w}_k^T \boldsymbol{x}_{ik} + b_k\right) \geq 1, \;\; i = 1, \ldots, s_k \text{ and } k = 1, \ldots, n$$

where s_k denotes the number of available samples from domain D_k. In this formulation we omit the slack variables included by [KZM+12] for simplification reasons and because they are unnecessary here for the further formulations. The parameter λ balances the influence of the global and the local models. Small values of λ lead to a high influence of the first term, thus in the course of optimization $w_g \rightarrow \mathbf{0}$ which means the local models are only weakly coupled. Vice versa, for $\lambda \rightarrow \infty$ this results in a regular linear SVM trained on the combined data from all domains. The optimization by stochastic sub-gradient descent is of no interest at this point, refer to [KZM$^+$12] for details. Previously unseen data from novel domains is processed by the global visual world model.

2.3 Large-margin dimension reduction

Face recognition is no closed-world two-class problem, but an open-world n-class problem where open-world means the number of classes is usually unknown. In most cases the question to be answered is if two samples belong to the same class, meaning: Do they show the same person? Let $z_i \in \mathbb{N}$ be the indicator variable that denotes the unique class-ID for each object, then

$$y_{ij} = \begin{cases} 1 & \text{, if } z_i = z_j \\ -1 & \text{, if } z_i \neq z_j \end{cases}$$

indicates if a sample pair shows the same person. One possibility to address this problem is by projecting the feature vectors into a discriminative target space where the distance between samples can be used to decide whether they are the same class [HB15a, SPVZ13]. In this case, the projection includes a dimension reduction based on the max-margin thought of SVMs. High dimensional features $\boldsymbol{\varphi}_i$ are projected to low dimensional features $\boldsymbol{v}_i$ by a projection matrix W

$$\boldsymbol{v}_i = W \boldsymbol{\varphi}_i$$

such that the squared euclidean distance $d^2(\boldsymbol{v}_i, \boldsymbol{v}_i) = d^2_W(\boldsymbol{\varphi}_i, \boldsymbol{\varphi}_j)$ in the target space is discriminative for face recognition tasks. Specifically, W should be chosen in a large-margin manner:

$$d^2_W(\boldsymbol{\varphi}_i, \boldsymbol{\varphi}_j) = (\boldsymbol{\varphi}_i - \boldsymbol{\varphi}_j)^T W^T W (\boldsymbol{\varphi}_i - \boldsymbol{\varphi}_j) \begin{cases} < b - 1 & \text{, if } y_{ij} = 1 \\ > b + 1 & \text{, if } y_{ij} = -1 \end{cases} \tag{2.5}$$

This forces the distance between samples of the same class to lie below the threshold b minus a margin and the distance between samples of different classes to lie above the threshold b plus a margin, as also shown in Fig. 2.3. Similar to the hinge-loss formulation of the linear SVM in equation (2.2), this can also be expressed as hinge-loss

$$l = \sum_{ij} \max\left(0, 1 - y_{ij} \cdot \left(b - d_W^2(\varphi_i, \varphi_j)\right)\right) \tag{2.6}$$

and a stochastic sub-gradient descent update of

$$W^{t+1} = \begin{cases} W^t & \text{, if } 1 - y_{ij} \cdot \left(b - d_W^2(\varphi_i, \varphi_j)\right) < 0 \\ W^t - \alpha y_{ij} W^t \Psi_{ij} & \text{, otherwise} \end{cases},$$

where

$$\Psi_{ij} = (\varphi_i - \varphi_j)(\varphi_i - \varphi_j)^T$$

and W^0 is initialized by a PCA.

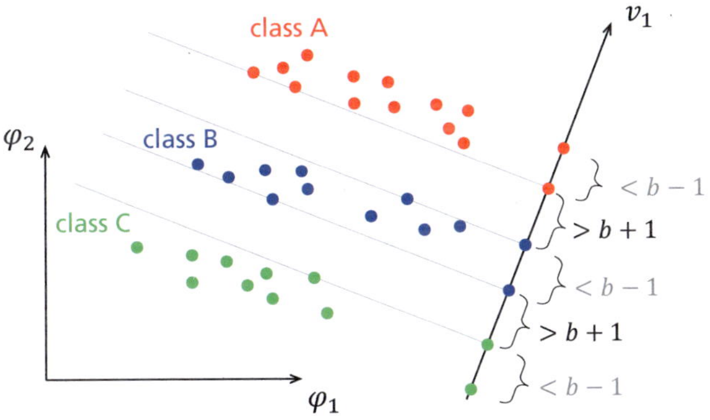

Figure 2.3: Visualization of the idea behind the max-margin dimension reduction strategy. The intra-class distances in the target space should be less than $b - 1$ while the inter-class distances should be larger than $b + 1$.

2.4 Large-margin dimension reduction with unsupervised domain adaptation

When analyzing the approach from [HB15a, SPVZ13], it becomes clear that the supervised dimension reduction step is responsible for possible domain dependencies. Consequently, a novel approach based on the combination of the unsupervised domain adaptation strategy presented in section 2.2 and the large-margin dimension reduction presented in the previous section, is proposed for the dimension reduction. First, we transfer the concept of local domain models from equation (2.3), which consist of a global visual world model and a bias, to the large-margin dimension reduction model:

$$\begin{aligned} W_k &= W_g + \Delta_k \\ b_k &= b_g + \delta_k. \end{aligned}$$

Because the model (W, b) consists of a projection matrix W and a threshold b, two bias components are necessary here, a bias matrix Δ_k and a scalar bias δ_k. Let φ_{ik} denote the i-th sample from the k-th domain, then the distances in the target space are

$$\begin{aligned} d_g\left(\varphi_{ik}, \varphi_{jk}\right) &= \left(\varphi_{ik} - \varphi_{jk}\right)^T W_g^T W_g \left(\varphi_{ik} - \varphi_{jk}\right) \\ d_k\left(\varphi_{ik}, \varphi_{jk}\right) &= \left(\varphi_{ik} - \varphi_{jk}\right)^T W_k^T W_k \left(\varphi_{ik} - \varphi_{jk}\right). \end{aligned}$$

The requirements regarding the thresholds b_g and b_k are analog to equation (2.5). Together with the equations (2.4) and (2.6), this leads to the hinge-loss formulation

$$\begin{aligned} l = &\sum_{i,j,k} max\left(0, 1 - y_{ijk}(b_g - d_g\left(\varphi_{ik}, \varphi_{jk}\right)\right) + \\ &\lambda \sum_{i,j,k} max\left(0, 1 - y_{ijk}(b_k - d_k\left(\varphi_{ik}, \varphi_{jk}\right)\right). \end{aligned}$$

Again, λ balances the influence of the global visual world and local domain models. For $\lambda = 0$ this collapses to the solution from equation (2.6) trained on the combined data from different domains.

Optimization is performed by a stochastic sub-gradient method. At each iteration sampling with equal frequency from each dataset and positive/negative samples. Given a pair of samples φ_{ik} and φ_{jk}, the updates are

$$\begin{aligned} W_g^{t+1} &= W_g^t - \alpha y_{ijk} W_g \Psi_{ijk} - \beta \lambda y_{ijk} W_k \Psi_{ijk} \\ \Delta_k^{t+1} &= \Delta_k^t - \beta \lambda y_{ijk} W_k \Psi_{ijk} \\ b_g^{t+1} &= b_g^t + y_{ijk} b_0 \\ \delta_k^{t+1} &= \delta_k^t + y_{ijk} b_0 \end{aligned}$$

where

$$\alpha = \begin{cases} 0 & \text{, if } y_{ijk}\left(b_g - d_g^2\left(\varphi_{ik}, \varphi_{jk}\right)\right) > 1 \\ \alpha_0 & \text{, otherwise} \end{cases},$$

$$\beta = \begin{cases} 0 & \text{, if } y_{ijk}\left(b_k - d_k^2\left(\varphi_{ik}, \varphi_{jk}\right)\right) > 1 \\ \beta_0 & \text{, otherwise} \end{cases} \quad \text{and}$$

$$\Psi_{ijk} = \left(\varphi_{ik} - \varphi_{jk}\right)\left(\varphi_{ik} - \varphi_{jk}\right)^T .$$

Both, α_0 and β_0 are arbitrary learning rates. Initialization for W_g^0 is performed by PCA and W_k^0 are initialized all zero. Finally, the local models (W_k, b_k) are discarded and the global model (W_g, b_g) which represents the whole visual world is kept for application on novel domains.

3 Conclusion

Two different strategies using the concept of a linear SVM were revisited, each solving one specific problem in terms of face recognition. The common underlying concept allowed a unified formulation, which includes both, a large-margin dimension reduction and an unsupervised domain adaptation. This method addresses the issue to better generalize from training data in order to build supervised face recognition applications that will also work well on previously unseen data.

Bibliography

[FHST13] Basura Fernando, Amaury Habrard, Marc Sebban, and Tinne Tuytelaars. Unsupervised visual domain adaptation using subspace alignment. In *Computer Vision (ICCV), 2013 IEEE International Conference on*, pages 2960–2967. IEEE, 2013.

[GLC11] Raghuraman Gopalan, Ruonan Li, and Rama Chellappa. Domain adaptation for object recognition: An unsupervised approach. In *Computer Vision (ICCV), 2011 IEEE International Conference on*, pages 999–1006. IEEE, 2011.

[HB15a] Christian Herrmann and Jürgen Beyerer. Face Retrieval on Large-Scale Video Data. In *Computer and Robot Vision*, pages 192–199, 2015.

[HRBLM07] Gary B. Huang, Manu Ramesh, Tamara Berg, and Erik Learned-Miller. Labeled Faces in the Wild: A Database for Studying Face Recognition in Unconstrained Environments. Technical Report 07-49, University of Massachusetts, Amherst, October 2007.

[KZM+12] Aditya Khosla, Tinghui Zhou, Tomasz Malisiewicz, Alexei Efros, and Antonio Torralba. Undoing the Damage of Dataset Bias. In *European Conference on Computer Vision*, Florence, Italy, October 2012.

[PGLC15] Vishal M Patel, Raghuraman Gopalan, Ruonan Li, and Rama Chellappa. Visual Domain Adaptation: A survey of recent advances. *Signal Processing Magazine, IEEE*, 32(3):53–69, 2015.

[QCSSL09] Joaquin Quionero-Candela, Masashi Sugiyama, Anton Schwaighofer, and Neil D Lawrence. *Dataset shift in machine learning*. The MIT Press, 2009.

[SPVZ13] Karen Simonyan, Omkar M Parkhi, Andrea Vedaldi, and Andrew Zisserman. Fisher vector faces in the wild. In *British Machine Vision Conference*, volume 1, page 7, 2013.

[TE+11] Antonio Torralba, Alexei Efros, et al. Unbiased look at dataset bias. In *Computer Vision and Pattern Recognition (CVPR), 2011 IEEE Conference on*, pages 1521–1528. IEEE, 2011.

[WHM11] L. Wolf, T. Hassner, and I. Maoz. Face recognition in unconstrained videos with matched background similarity. In *Computer Vision and Pattern Recognition*, 2011.

Considerations on Trajectory Planning Models in Automated Driving

Miriam Ruf

Fraunhofer IOSB,
Karlsruhe, Germany
miriam.ruf@iosb.fraunhofer.de

Technical Report IES-2015-04

Abstract: The SPARC concept for fully-automated driving was introduced in 2012 as a way to overcome the highly discretized maneuver planning approaches that had previously dominated the DARPA Grand and Urban Challenges. The aim was to define a single planner that is responsible for all forward driving tasks, including intersections, highways and pre-crash situations; that is based on a sound statistical framework including prediction and sensing uncertainties; and that can trade off between goals like safety, comfort and efficiency in a unified and transparent way. Since then, several similar approaches have been presented, most notably the Bertha Benz drive of 2013, in which the 100 km distance between Mannheim and Pforzheim was covered autonomously in a Mercedes–Benz S-500 Intelligent Drive. During the same time, the SPARC approach has been refined in several respects, including its vehicle models and optimization techniques. This technical report provides an overview of the avenues explored to motivate the current form of the SPARC concept, based on frequently-asked questions that arose during the various technical presentations of the concept.

1 Background and Motivation of SPARC

The SPARC (Situation Prediction and Reacting Control) concept (introduced in [Zie12, RZR⁺14]) was created within the V50 project aimed at developing solutions for fully-automated inner-city driving; the specific task assigned to Fraunhofer IOSB was to provide two modules – situation detection and maneuver planning. The project structure is shown in Fig. 1.1. The approach was chosen to overcome drawbacks with highly discretized approaches that were commonly used previously to this and, for example, dominated the DARPA Grand

and Urban Challenges (cf. [RZR+14]). Examples include the use of discrete velocity profiles for the ego vehicle [UAB+08], discrete "situation states" in which the ego vehicle can be [MBB+08, CSA+09], or arbitrating the responsibility for the driving task dynamically between various dedicated planning systems [UAB+08, MBB+08, WSM09, BBF+08]. The goal of SPARC was to express all driving tasks in a unified ("holistic") way, governed by a universal set of rules that remains constant from parking to pre-crash, and from urban intersections to interstate highways.

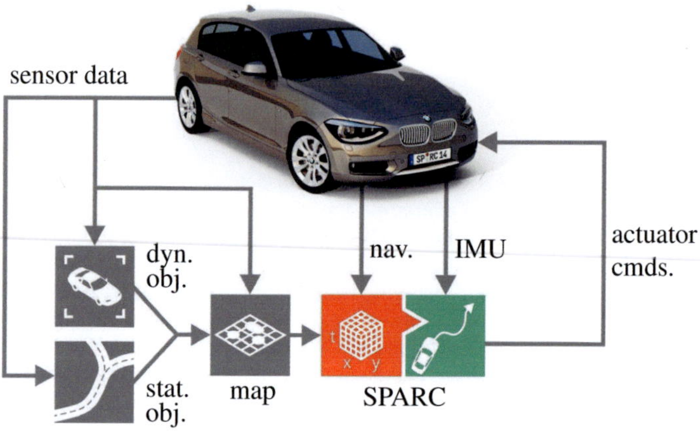

Figure 1.1: Overview of the V50 project. Sensor data is processed to detect dynamic objects (cars, pedestrians, cyclists, ...) and static objects (walls, signs, traffic lights, roads, road markings, ...) in the environment. The information is combined in a dynamic map, which presents the basis for SPARC. The Situation Prediction (SP, red) stage predicts the future development of the scene, determines applicable traffic rules and sets waypoints based on navigation instructions. The Reaction Control (RC, green) stage uses this information to compute an optimal trajectory and execute it using the actuators (steering, acceleration, lights, ...).

The SPARC module receives information from a *dynamic map* of tracked static and dynamic objects and features detected in the vicinity of the ego vehicle. The *Situation Prediction* (SP) stage predicts the behavior of dynamic objects into the near future (5–10 seconds), and estimates for each object at every (future) time step the severity of a possible collision (cf. [RZW+14a]). It also determines applicable traffic rules (such as speed limits, overtaking rules or stop signs) and assigns penalties to their violation. Finally it uses navigation instructions to set coarse waypoints for the ego vehicle. All of this information is passed to the *Reaction Control* (RC) stage, which uses it to plan an optimal trajectory for the ego vehicle to the proximity of the waypoints, by minimizing collision risks, traffic rule violations, passenger inconvenience, fuel consumption and wear of vehicle parts ([RZR$^+$14, RZW$^+$15]). The earliest control inputs of the optimized maneuver are passed to the vehicle actuators.

This process is repeated at a rate of 10 Hz, so that the planning horizon of the trajectory does not just cover the gap between updates, but assures that the currently executed actuator commands are part of a long-term plan that is considered safe by the currently best prediction. Any unforeseen developments will be accounted for in the following update.

Should the environment predictions not be updated due to a significant system failure (e.g. sensor blackout or crash of the SP stage), during each cycle, the RC stage also computes a fail-safe emergency trajectory that is also based on the same predictions but will not lead the ego vehicle to the next waypoint, but to a safe place on the side of the road (see [RZW$^+$15] for details).

Since the original publications [Zie12, RZR$^+$14], several similar approaches have been presented, most notably [ZBDS14], which successfully completed the fully-automated 100 km Bertha-Benz drive from Mannheim to Pforzheim in 2013. Despite using equivalent models with a similar motivation, the SPARC approach is unique in several design decisions that have aroused some discussion during previous presentations, and shall thus be motivated in the following sections with particular respect to possible alternatives.

2 Model Decisions in SPARC

This section will motivate key decisions and discuss alternatives related to two main areas of SPARC: The problem formulation over predicted, expected risks traded off against comfort, ecology and traffic rule compliance, integrated in an Euler-Lagrange model (Sec. 2.1); and the optimization of this Euler-Lagrange model through a Hidden Markov Model, instead of an iterative solver (Sec. 2.2).

2.1 Use of Expected Risks and the Euler-Lagrange Model

The most basic motivation of the SPARC approach was to define an evaluation *functional* $\mathcal{H}[\xi]$ that maps a given trajectory $\xi(t)$ onto non-negative real numbers, such that the most desired functions $\overset{*}{\xi}(t)$ are recognized by having assigned the least $\mathcal{H}[\xi^*]$. This section will present the choice of $\mathcal{H}$, the alternatives considered, and the rationale behind the eventual choice.

To embed SPARC into well-developed theoretical frameworks, two key features were considered relevant: Additivity and a stochastic foundation. These two individual properties, along with the combination as *additive stochastic models*, will be motivated and illustrated in this section.

Additivity An evaluation functional based exclusively on a function H whose value is additive

$$\mathcal{H}[\xi] = \int_{t_\text{start}}^{t_\text{end}} \mathrm{d}t \; H(\xi(t), \dot{\xi}(t), \ddot{\xi}(t), ..., \tfrac{\mathrm{d}^n}{\mathrm{d}t^n}\xi(t), t) \tag{2.1}$$

restricts the expressiveness of $\mathcal{H}$ considerably. Its application is limited to $\xi \in C^n$, and it is impossible to model long-term dependencies, such as requiring that ξ have exactly three roots. It is also impossible to evaluate a dynamic range of derivatives, such as requiring that ξ have an arbitrarily great but even number of nonzero derivatives at each point.

These limitations however bring about a significant advantage: It originally arose from the physical study of particle trajectories, both for photons and matter, and therefore has been studied extensively. A particularly relevant result is the Euler-Lagrange equation [VB10], which provides an efficiently computable necessary criterion for the optimality of a trajectory $\xi^{\circledast}$, namely

$$\delta_\xi \mathcal{H} := \frac{\partial H}{\partial \xi} - \frac{\mathrm{d}}{\mathrm{d}t}\frac{\partial H}{\partial \dot{\xi}} + ... + (-1)^n \frac{\mathrm{d}^n}{\mathrm{d}t^n}\frac{\partial H}{\partial \frac{\mathrm{d}^n}{\mathrm{d}t^n}\xi}, \tag{2.2}$$

such that, if $\xi^{\circledast}$ is optimal, $\delta_\xi \mathcal{H}\big|_{\xi^{\circledast}} \equiv 0$, which allows to find solutions analytically. In numerical solutions of (2.1), where ξ is a vector in $\mathbb{R}^{\#t}$ over $\#t$ discrete time steps, $\delta_\xi \mathcal{H}$ takes the role of a gradient (in fact, [ZRR+15] shows that (2.2) can be derived directly as a gradient) that can be used to iteratively optimize from an "initial guess" $\xi^{(0)}$ towards a local optimum ξ^*. At the same time, this formulation of $\mathcal{H}$ allows to cover a wide range of optimality criteria that arise in (automated) driving situations, namely

- Safety, by penalizing combinations of ξ and t that represent a possible future collision with another traffic participant, or lane departures.
- Comfort and ecology, by penalizing strong accelerations $\ddot{\xi}$ and jerks $\dddot{\xi}$.
- Traffic rule compliance, e.g. by penalizing exceeding speed limits via $\dot{\xi}$.

Furthermore, [RZW+14b] shows that a significant number of vehicle parameters, such as wheel speeds and steering wheel angles, can be analytically expressed in terms of derivatives, and are thus available for use in H. These parameters can be used inside an Euler-Lagrange model (ELM) if lateral and longitudinal wheel slip are not considered.[1] Simulation results presented therein show, that even under highly dynamic conditions, these simplifications (necessary to make the vehicle model compatible with the ELM) provide a good approximation to the actual vehicle behavior (cf. Fig. 2.1).

Additionally, various types of *boundary conditions* can be added to express properties of ξ at t_{start} and t_{end}, in particular constraining ξ to the current vehicle position at t_{start} and penalizing deviations from a goal position at t_{end}. The only key limitation that remains is that all time instances of ξ must be evaluated independently through H, so that non-local dependencies between any values attained by ξ cannot be modeled.

Stochastical Models Most established mathematical models in artificial intelligence-related fields are equipped with a stochastic interpretation. While their computation often relies heavily on simplifications to preserve tractability (such as the assumption of conditional independence), all simplifications can be made explicit, and thus can be validated or falsified in comparision with real-world statistics. The stochastic interpretation also provides a convenient way of combining different models on a well-understood basis. On the other hand, models that circumvent stochastic modeling are usually less easily analyzed in terms of assumptions and quality of results, and thus less easily combined. For fully-automated driving, the main aspects to be combined through stochastical modeling are:

[1] Estimating the current and future grip of a vehicle under practical driving conditions is considered a highly difficult problem. Therefore, any predicted grip value would likely be speculative anyway.

- Sensor uncertainties (such as noise, blur and occlusion)
- Sensor processing uncertainties (e.g., remaining classification ambiguity)
- Prediction uncertainty (such as uncertain lane changes in other cars)
- Actuator uncertainty (such as unknown friction for a braking maneuver)

Stochastical models must thus be found that both allow to express these uncertainties and fit the limitations of the ELM (2.1).

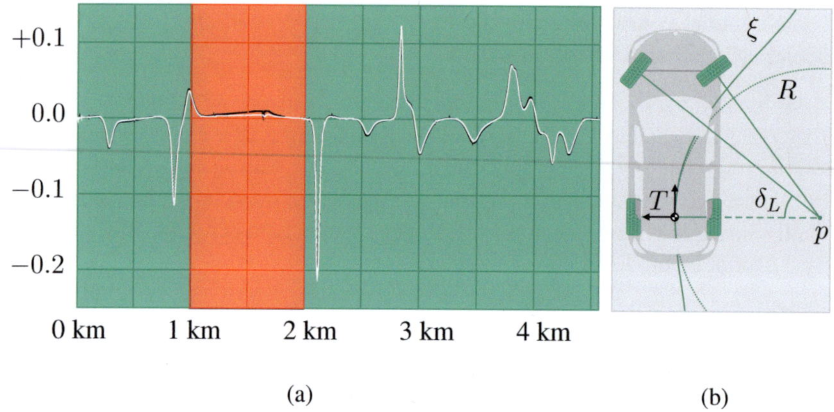

Figure 2.1: The C^2 model presented in [RZW$^+$14b]. (a) Estimated steering wheel angles (white) compared to steering wheel angles obtained in a state-of-the-art physical simulation of the Hockenheimring race track (black). The red section shows deviations during to lateral slip in a bend driven at 170 km/h. Everywhere else, the estimations of the C^2 model match the simulation closely. (b) The geometry of the C^2 model is based on the tangent coordinate system T of the trajectory ξ, and its circle of curvature R centered at p. This allows to describe a multi-track vehicle with Ackermann steering; the left wheel angle δ_L is indicated.

Additive Stochastic Models The two most prominent stochastic models that aim or allow for additivity are log-linear models and independent expected values, both of which rely on assumptions of stochastic independence. We will introduce stochastic independence, and briefly discuss log-linear models, to motivate why expected values were instead preferred for the use in SPARC.

Probabilities that are stochastically independent can be multiplied to obtain the joint probability. A common example is the cast of two dice. Both dice have a probability $p(d\!=\!n) = 1/6,\ n\!\in\!\{1,...,6\}$ of rolling an "n". The probability of one dice rolling a 1, the other a 6, is given as $p(d_1\!=\!1 \wedge d_2\!=\!6)\!=\!p(d_1\!=\!1)\cdot p(d_2\!=\!6)\!=\!1/36$ by virtue of the assumption of stochastic independence; the cast of either dice is not expected to influence the other. A counterexample is rolling a *single* dice *once*, and giving the probability of the *same* dice producing both values in a single cast ($p(d_1 = 1 \wedge d_1 = 6)$). While both individual probabilities remain $1/6$, their joint probability is 0 – the results are not independent, as one will strictly rule out the other.

More often than not in practical applications, stochastic independence is taken as a convenient simplification rather than the true system behavior. For example, motion tracking algorithms may describe their next target motions as independent from previously observed motions, while in most cases the targets are *known* to not act randomly. However, this assumption allows each timestep to be treated in a uniform fashion, and the corresponding models can be more easily parametrized since complex and long-term behavior patterns can be ignored, and individual transition probabilities can be multiplied repeatedly over time to obtain the probability distribution of future locations.

Log-linear models are based on the realization that this multiplicative accumulation corresponds to an additive accumulation in the space of logarithmic proabilities:

$$\log\left(\prod_{n\in N} p_n\right) = \sum_{n\in N} \log(p_n)$$

Thus by taking the logarithm of each probability, a quantity is obtained that can be summed while retaining the stochastic interpretation in the result. The stochastic model is said to be *log-linear*. In this way, models that rely exclusively on probabilities can be subject to linear optimization, usually to *maximize probabilities*.

However, many applications cannot be adequately modeled through probabilities. It stands to reason that automotive traffic (or locomotion in general) is not intuitively a pure maximation or minimization of probabilities. While occasionally argued, a desirable trajectory is not that which minimizes the probability of an accident, since this trajectory would in most cases remain stationary forever and not even attempt to reach a faraway destination. We can further conceive the case of a pre-crash situation, where the driver can choose between a certain ($p_1 = 1$) rear-end collision with the car in front of him at low speed, or taking an evasive maneuver to the opposite lane and stopping the car amid oncoming traffic. The probability of an accident is "worst" for the rear-end collision, yet this option will usually be preferred to the lower but more severe risk of colliding with oncoming cars at high speed.

The key alternative thus appears to be *risk*, used here as the *expected value of detriment*, however the latter may be defined. For illustration purposes only we can consider the *detriment* H of a collision as given purely by the costs of the damage, which for the low-speed rear-end collision may be $H_1 = \$5\,000$, while a high-speed head-on collision may cost $H_2 = \$100\,000$. Now considering a $p_2 = 1/10$ chance of colliding with oncoming traffic, we have an expected cost of $p_1 \cdot H_1 = \$5\,000$ for the rear-end collision (which is, as stated, certain), and $p_2 \cdot H_2 = \$10\,000$ for the head-on collision, which is considerably higher.

Let us assume that in this case the driver chooses to accept the rear-end collision, but finds himself in almost the same situation on the same road one month later. The collision costs remain the same, but this time he evades to the opposite lane.

Now we can expect the total damage arising from these two situations to be $p_1 \cdot H_1 + p_2 \cdot H_2 = \$15\,000$. We realize that the expected costs were *added*, based on the intuition that the outcomes of the two accidents are independent. But are they?

Not strictly: Had the driver decided differently, and collided with an oncoming car in the first case, the damaged car is less likely to be repaired by then, and thus the collision risk is lower since one possible collision partner is missing. The outcomes are not independent, but considering the sheer number of possible collision partners, the dependence is slight and difficult to model. Whether or not expected values can be added thus also relies on stochastic independence, and whether or not possible dependencies (as in this case) must be included in the model depends on an understanding of the model.

What is gained by modeling with expected values, however, is the inclusion of two parameters – the detriment and the probability – which provides a bridge between pure probabilities and their real-world implications. Once a unit for detriment (here the costs in \$) has been set, stochastic events (such as collisions) and deterministic events (such as detriment from high fuel consumption or uncomfortable accelerations) can be directly compared: What makes human drivers accept risks that are inherent to participating in road traffic is a trade-off between the risks and the gains. For example, human drivers pass pedestrians on the side-walk even if there is a risk of them jumping onto the road before them in the last second; the probability is considered extremely low and the detriment of braking to walking speed before passing any pedestrian is considerable in terms of travel time and fuel consumption.

Using expected values, these trade-offs, that are implicit to human driving can be rendered explicit and quantitative for automated driving. Details on how the predicted occupancy probabilities of other traffic participants are obtained can be found in [RZW+14a].

2.2 Local vs. Global Optimization

Given a functional based on the previous criteria, the optimization goal

$$\xi^* = \arg\min_{\xi} H[\xi]$$

uniquely identifies a trajectory or a set of trajectories which are, based on the model, of indistinguishable quality. Obtaining a minimal element, however, is not trivial. The most commonly used method for optimization, an iterative descent such as a gradient descent or extensions of Newton's method (SQP, BFGS, L-BFGS), are risky to apply in automated driving, for reasons that will be detailed in this section based on [RZW+15]. An alternative model is outlined that mitigates these risks while retaining real-time capability.

2.2.1 Risks Associated to Iterative Optimization

Iterative solvers start from an "initial guess" $\xi^{(0)}$, and apply an optimization step $\xi^{(n-1)} \mapsto \xi^{(n)}$, usually with the goal that $H[\xi^{(n)}] < H[\xi^{(n-1)}]$. The process terminates based on criteria for $\xi^{(n)}$, and possibly n, $\xi^{(n-1)}$ and other properties. Common termination criteria are

$$\begin{aligned} H[\xi^{(n)}] &< T_A && \text{(sufficiently low value)} \\ |H[\xi^{(n)}] - H[\xi^{(n-1)}]| &< T_B && \text{(sufficiently small value step)} \\ \left.\frac{\mathrm{d}H}{\mathrm{d}\xi}\right|_{\xi^{(n)}} &< T_C && \text{(sufficiently small gradient)} \\ n &> N && \text{(computation time exhausted)} \end{aligned}$$

The main problems associated with this are already apparent from the above formulation. Firstly, none of the above uses truly *global* properties, i.e. the relation of $\xi^{(n)}$ to arbitrary other members of the function space. At best, a small subset of dimension 1 is evaluated. Thus, the process can terminate in a stationary point or local optimum that is far from the global optimum. Secondly, not even local convergence can be strictly measured, but is given in terms of thresholds. Thus, the process can terminate even in points that are not stationary, but merely too slightly sloped. Thirdly, the process can terminate after a fixed number N of iterations disregarding *any* properties that $\xi^{(N)}$ might hold – or run an arbitrarily long time.[2]

In total, it can be said that properties of the obtained solution $\tilde{\xi}^*$ are difficult to predict. Beside the problem structure (which is the only desirable influence), they depend significantly on the initial guess and the optimization step; in many cases, these even dominate the solution. The influence is generally *not* intuitive, as $\xi^{(0)}$ will not necessarily converge to (e.g.) the closest local optimum, or the optimum towards which the first gradient points.

This uncertainty about thc quality of the optimization result, combined with the possibility of strongly varying optimization times, suggests a high risk of applying local iterative optimization to high-risk real-time applications such as automated driving. Examples of all of the above claims, arising in simple, everyday traffic situations, will be given in detail in an upcoming publication.

2.2.2 Strategies to Improve Iterated Optimization

One method considered as a candidate for the generation of initial guesses is the partition of the planning space by Voronoi lines between local risk maxima.

As used here, a (Euclidean) Voronoi diagram on a space $\Sigma \subseteq \mathbb{R}^n$, based on a finite set $P \subset \Sigma$ of points, partitions Σ into *cells* C such that $|P| = |C|$,

$$\sigma \in c_i \quad \Longleftarrow \quad p_i \in \arg\min_{p \in P} \|p - \sigma\|_2$$

which implies

$$\bigcup_{c \in C} c = \Sigma$$

2 It should also be noted that divergence can take many different forms, from infinite loops over increasingly bad solutions up to chaotic behavior. It is thus difficult to detect and even harder to resolve.

but also provides

$$V = \bigcup_{c',c'' \in C} c' \cap c''$$

such that for $|P| > 1$ and a convex Σ it holds[3] that $V \neq \emptyset$ and $\dim(V) = \dim(\Sigma) - 1$. We also introduce a finite set

$$I = \{v \in V \mid \exists c', c'', c''' \in C : v = c' \cap c'' \cap c'''\}$$

of *intersections* in V, i.e. points at which at least three cells intersect.

For a two-dimensional risk field $H_R : X \times T \to \mathbb{R}$, a Voronoi diagram between the local maxima of H_R provides a one-dimensional V, which resembles a lattice of lines over $X \times T$ between the local maxima, as shown in Fig. 2.3. As these lines avoid local maxima of H_R, they can be used to provide initial guesses for trajectories $\xi : T \to X$. A straightforward approach would be to perform a graph search by using the elements of I as nodes in a graph G, with edges denoting direct connections in V. Then paths in G can be used to hint at initial guesses for ξ^*.

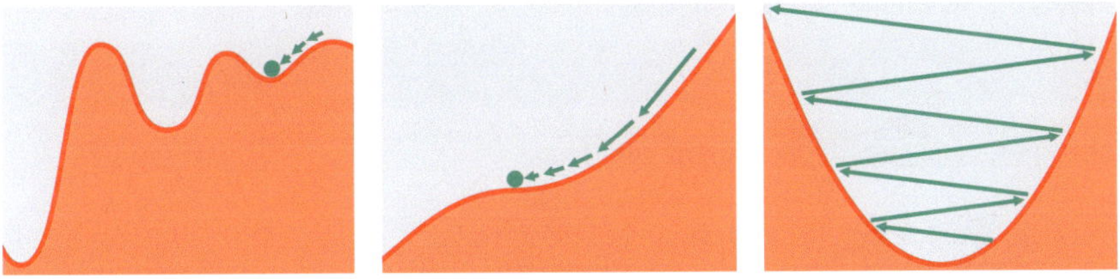

(a) Local optimum (b) Stationary point (c) Divergence

Figure 2.2: Increasingly undesirable convergence behaviors of an iterative solver. (a) The solver converges to a local optimum that is considerably worse than the global optimum. (b) The solver converges to a stationary point instead of any optimum. (c) The solver does not converge at all. Each case can occur under realistic conditions; in real-time high-risk scenarios, the consequences can be serious.

[3] Proof: As $|P| > 1$ (and finite) then $\forall p_1 \in \Sigma\ \exists p_2 \in \Sigma$ s.t. $p_2 \in \arg\min_{p \in P} \|p_1 - p\|_2$. Then, as Σ is convex, $\exists \sigma_m = (p_1 + p_2)/2 \in \Sigma$; also $\arg\min_{p \in P} \|p - \sigma_m\|_2 \supseteq \{p_1, p_2\}$. Thus $\sigma_m \in V$.

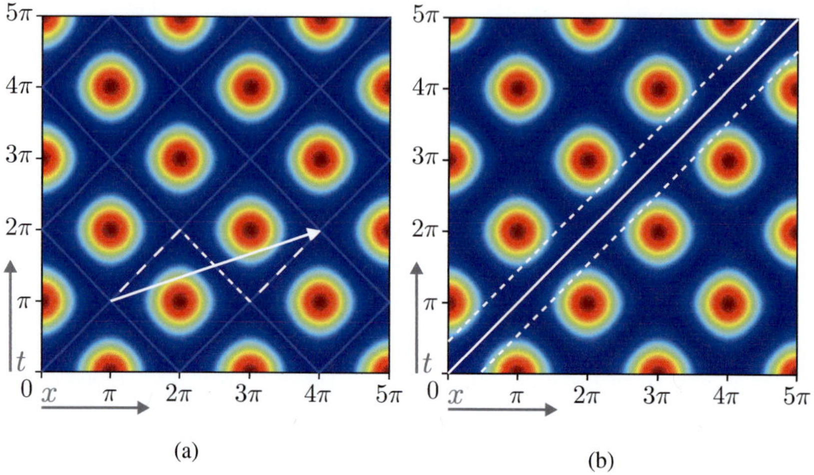

Figure 2.3: Inabilities in the Voronoi enumerating the local optima. (a) V (light blue) and a path through G (white dashed, dotted) using an edge backward through time (dotted) that would be omitted. No valid connection in G between source and goal point exists, even though there is a potential local optimum (arrow). (b) Effect of some $\alpha > 0$ (weighting factor of some goal speed) limiting even all *local* optima to within the dashed band of width $2d$. The Voronoi diagram cannot account for this limitation.

This, however, entails a series of problems:

- V does not generally include the point in $X \times T$ that is considered the initial position of the vehicle $\xi(0)$. Thus a new connection between $\xi(0)$ and V must be created that is difficult to motivate within the model.
- Paths in G can move backwards through time. These cases can and must be excluded, but this issue hints at a deeper problem:
- Paths in G are based on geometric considerations that consider the two space dimensions as interchangeable. Therefore, temporal distances and spatial distances are considered equal, which requires the choice of a conversion factor. This factor determines the solution (cf. Fig. 2.5) even though it is unlikely to stem from any physical motivation. In this case, the number of free parameters, that are not motivated through the problem, increases. This is generally undesirable, as these parameters are not easily adapted to changes in the problem.

- Paths in G depend exclusively on the structure of H_R but have generally no relation to, for example, the dynamical model of the vehicle or target positions, speeds and accelerations. Thus, in particular the notion of locality can differ significantly: The basically possible paths through V (moving forward through time, respecting speed limits, ...) do *not* enumerate the local optima of $\mathcal{H}[\xi]$ since $\mathcal{H}[\xi]$ has a (significantly) higher dimension than H_R, and this dimension is highly relevant, as can be seen in the following examples:

  - Additional local optima can arise from penalties on, e.g., speeds, that cannot be derived from H_R. Fig. 2.3 gives an example where significant local optima would be missed this way.
  - When paths "backwards in time" are simply removed, possible local optima are ignored, since V does *not* consider the "best" path between the optima in terms of the optimization functional, but the one with the highest space-time distance regardless of physical possibility. Consider the risk field[4]

    $$H_R(x,t) = (\cos(x) - \cos(t))^2, \quad x \in [0, 5\pi], t \in [0, 5\pi] \tag{2.3}$$

    Then $i_1 = [\pi, \pi]^T, i_2 = [2\pi, 2\pi]^T, i_3 = [3\pi, \pi]^T, i_4 = [4\pi, 2\pi]^T$ with $i_1, i_2, i_3, i_4 \in I$, but no edge between i_1 and i_4. There exists a path $i_1 \to i_2 \to i_3 \to i_4$, but this is not physically possible since $i_2 \to i_3$ moves backwards in time. It would thus naïvely be discarded, but (unlike in other similar cases, which are discarded rightfully) there exists a potentially locally optimal direct path connecting i_1 and i_4 that is physically possible and avoids all local maxima (albeit not at the furthest possible distance).
  - It is even possible that the number of local optima is *lower* than the paths through V. Consider again Fig. 2.3 and H_R as in (2.3), combined with the Lagrangian

    $$H(\xi, \dot{\xi}, t) = H_R(\xi, t) + \alpha \cdot (\dot{\xi} - 1)^2, \quad \alpha > 0$$

    which penalizes, in addition to H_R, deviations from the goal speed of $\dot{\xi} = 1$, weighted by α. Analytically we obtain the Euler-Lagrange

[4] And do notice that the lack of physical dimensions is not the fault of the example, but rather symptomatic of what a purely geometric model allows and, in a sense, requires.

equation as

$$\underbrace{2\sin(\xi)\big(\cos(t)-\cos(\xi)\big)}_{A} - \underbrace{\alpha\cdot\ddot{\xi}}_{B} \equiv 0 \tag{2.4}$$

which is, for the boundary conditions $\xi(0)=0,\ \dot{\xi}(0)=1,\ \xi(5\pi)=5\pi$, trivially satisfied for $\xi^*(t) = t$, a global optimum regardless of the choice of α, as $\mathcal{H} \geq 0$ and here $\mathcal{H} = 0$. Other local optima may exist that also satisfy (2.4). However there exists some α_T such that for any $\alpha > \alpha_\mathrm{T}$, all local optima but the global optimum vanish. This can be proven by contradiction.

Assume there exists some $\xi^{\circledast} \not\equiv \xi^*$ such that (2.4) is satisfied, so there exists $t \in T$ and some $d \neq 0$ such that $\xi^{\circledast}(t) - \xi^*(t) = d$.

Reaching a given d within T from the fixed starting point requires an acceleration of $|\ddot{\xi}^{\circledast}(t)| > |4d/25\pi^2|$ at some instant t,[5] and thus, in (2.4), $|\alpha 4d/25\pi^2| < |B|$, presenting a lower bound for $|B|$ given α and d. In turn, A of (2.4) lies strictly within $[-3\sqrt{3}/2, +3\sqrt{3}/2]$. For $A - B$ to vanish, it is thus necessary that

$$\min|B| \leq \max|A| \Rightarrow \left|\alpha\frac{4d}{25\pi^2}\right| \leq \left|\frac{3\sqrt{3}}{2}\right| \Rightarrow |d| \leq \frac{75\sqrt{3}\pi^2}{8\alpha}$$

Intuitively, to reach a larger d (given α), there exists at least one $B(t)$ so great that no position gradient $A(\xi, t)$ can outweigh it to satisfy (2.4). Thus for large α, $|d|$ can be forced arbitrarily small, limiting any $\xi^{\circledast}$ to $|\xi^* - \xi^{\circledast}| \leq d$. Solutions outside this band are impossible, but present valid paths in G, as it is based exclusively on H_R and does not vary with α. Thus, while the choice of α can reduce the number of local optima down to 1, the number of paths in G is invariant to α.

There is no obvious way to remedy these issues: The practical disadvantages of the Voronoi approach lie in the fact that it treats space and time as equivalent (and not in a relativistic sense) and cannot account for vehicle dynamics – which are a significant part of the topology of the trajectory space. Extending the dimensionality of V so that it is not based on H_R alone, but on the abstract trajectory space Ξ, is generally possible; however, building a Voronoi diagram in Ξ requires

[5] In fact, only when applied during *all* t this acceleration achieves d; and only at t_end, not the true goal point. Thus the inequality marks no *tight* lower bound, just some definitive lower bound. Any valid $\xi^{\circledast}$ visiting $\xi^{\circledast}(t') = t' \pm d$ and returning to $\xi(5\pi) = 5\pi$ would even require a higher acceleration.

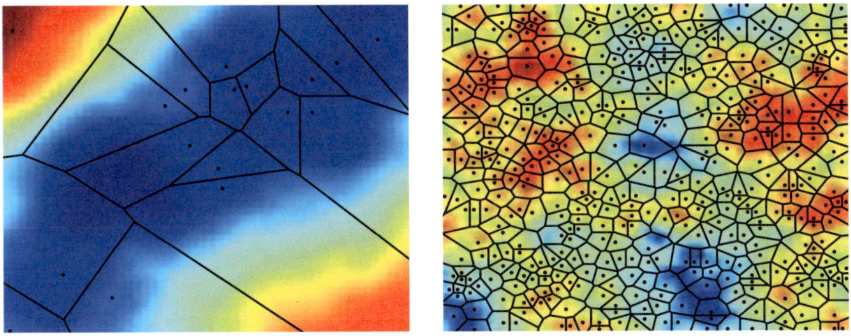

(a) $\gamma = 2.5$ (b) $\gamma = 1.5$

Figure 2.4: Brownian noise fields with different power spectrum distributions $S(\omega) \propto \omega^{-\gamma}$ (color map), local maxima (dots) and corresponding V (lines). Assuming (as used throughout this paper) the current position to be the lower left corner, it must be noted that V does not include this point. Next, in (a), V does not provide a path to the upper right corner even though it is intuitively desirable. In (b), V is a highly complex structure including many intersections and many paths along high H_R values. A valuable reduction of complexity with respect to the original pixel grid is not apparent.

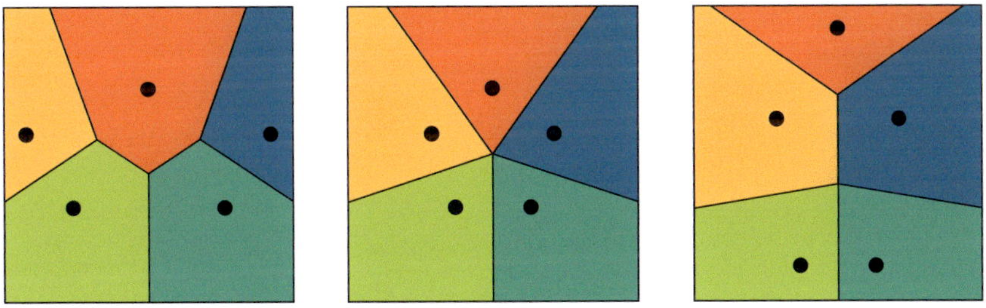

(a) (b) (c)

Figure 2.5: Voronoi diagrams for different aspect ratios between the horizontal and the vertical axis. It can be seen that the resulting topology differs in each case. If the axes represent different physical quantities, as time and space, this means that the solution is not invariant to the choice of units.

finding the local maxima, which corresponds to enumerating all *worst* trajectories in Ξ. If this initial step was efficiently possible, one could simply reverse the problem to enumerate all the *best* trajectories, and pick the global optimum directly, without the additional step of creating and searching a Voronoi diagram.

On the whole, while the paths through the Voronoi diagram certainly correlate with the true local optima, they provide neither an upper nor a lower bound. It was shown that the assumptions governing the Voronoi solution are not sound within the original model; therefore, extensive post-processing is necessary to make the Voronoi solutions even just valid *candidates* for the original model; in particular, a significant part of solutions must be discarded as they are physically impossible. Given all its inaccuracy, setting up and searching the Voronoi graph is anything but simple for complex environments (see Fig. 2.4). While eliminating the free parameter of $\xi^{(0)}$ (the "initial guess"), the Voronoi diagram introduces at least one new free parameter (the relative scale of time and space) that has an even less intuitive effect on the solution; further free parameters lie in how the obtained solutions are discarded or transformed into valid solutions of the ELM. For these reasons, the Voronoi approach was abandoned in favor of a solution that would both retain the key model features throughout the solution process (as, for example, the distinction between time and space), and that would provide clear algorithmic properties (computational effort and quality of results) to be compared with the previous ELM.

2.2.3 Global Optimization

The previous considerations suggest that iterative optimization is generally not able to guarantee the quality of a solution, or that it is found in limited time. Any obtained solution depends critically on parameters that cannot be determined by the problem understanding alone.

In this section, an approach to *global* optimization that provides *global* optima in finite time to the given problem will be presented. It can help address the issues with iterative optimization in two ways. First of all, the obtained global optimum can be used directly in maneuver planning. However, global optimization of sufficiently general problems comes at a price in computational effort, that may exceed either real-time constraints or acceptable hardware costs. Should global optimization prove too costly for real-time series integration (which has not been established yet, since this section will shed light on significant parallelization potential), global optimization can still provide benchmarks for iterative solvers, in the sense that previously, the true global solution of such a problem was not known at all, and thus the evaluation of iterative solvers had to rely on comparing different iterative solutions to each other.

To address the named pitfalls of iterative optimization without abandoning key properties of the original model, an approach based on [ZRR$^+$15] is chosen: The ELM is transformed into an equivalent Hidden Markov Model (HMM) such that, given a sufficiently fine discretization,

1. Globally optimal trajectories of the ELM correspond directly to the globally optimal state sequence attained by decoding the HMM through the Viterbi algorithm.
2. Values of $H[\xi]$ are provided a one-to-one mapping to sequence probabilities, such that in particular $H[\xi^*]$ can be obtained.

[ZRR$^+$15] shows that an ELM, whose Lagrangian can be separated into

$$H(\xi, \dot{\xi}, t) = H_1(x, t) + H_2(x, \dot{x}),$$

can be transformed into an equivalent HMM by choosing sufficiently fine discretizations $X' = \{x_{\text{min}}, x_{\text{min}} + \Delta x, x_{\text{min}} + 2\Delta x, ..., x_{\text{min}} + n\Delta x\}$ $(x_1 \in X)$ and $T' = \{t_{\text{start}}, t_{\text{start}} + \Delta t, t_{\text{start}} + 2\Delta t, ..., t_{\text{start}} + m\Delta t\}$ and choosing emission probabilities $p(\sigma_\tau | x_2)$ and transition probabilities $p(x_2 \leftarrow x_1 | x_1)$ as follows

$$\begin{aligned} p(\sigma_\tau | x_2) &= \frac{1}{Z_1} \cdot \exp(-H_1(x_2, \tau \cdot \Delta t + t_{\text{start}})) \\ p(x_2 \leftarrow x_1 | x_1) &= \frac{1}{Z_2} \cdot \exp(-H_2(x_2, \tfrac{x_2 - x_1}{\Delta t})) \end{aligned}$$

where the normalization constants Z_1 and Z_2 are uniquely defined. The correspondence in [ZRR$^+$15] extends to more general cases, but the above formulation was found sufficient to represent the SPARC approach for generalized coordinates including first-order derivatives. This transformation allows to apply the Viterbi algorithm, which determines the optimal sequence of states in X' over time T' within a fixed space of memory and in a fixed number of time steps:

$$\mathsf{VITERBI} \in \mathsf{TIME}(T' \cdot |X'|^2) \cap \mathsf{SPACE}(T' \cdot |X'|).$$

This can be contrasted with the computational complexity of iteratively solving the original ELM with a gradient descent (EL^1) or a variant of SQP using a full Hessian (EL^2), which can be written as

$$\mathsf{EL}^1 \in \mathsf{SPACE}(T') \quad \text{and} \quad \mathsf{EL}^2 \in \mathsf{SPACE}(T'^2),$$

if convergence occurs – however there is no limit on the TIME complexity, as arbitrarily many iterations can be required until then, and divergence (an infinite number of steps) may occur as well.

So, the HMM formulation addresses several key issues of the iterative optimization, namely:

- The HMM formulation does not require an "initial guess", an iteration step function $\xi^{(n)} \mapsto \xi^{(n+1)}$ or termination criteria as presented in Sec. 2.2.1. Their role as free parameters is replaced by the choice of a discretization Δx, which is considered considerably more intuitive in its results (cf. [ZRR$^+$15, RZW$^+$15]).
- The HMM solution through the Viterbi algorithm cannot diverge or require an arbitrary number of computation steps; instead, the solution is known to be found after a fixed number of computations.
- The Viterbi algorithm cannot get stuck in undesirable local optima. Its result is always the global optimum given the discretization, which does not directly equal the continuous global optimum, but is considerably less sensitive to parameters and the shape of the underlying problem $\mathcal{H}$.

Despite this, it can be said that on average, the HMM optimization requires more computations to finish than a gradient descent or SQP, and it scales particularly badly with the state space X', such that optimizing a pure two-dimensional path can already be prohibitively expensive ([RZW$^+$15] provides an adequate choice of X' that limits the computational effort while retaining sufficient expressiveness to model a multilane road).

However, comparing the number of necessary computations can be misleading, as parallelization can be a significant factor. For the ELM, the parallelization dimension is T', since for a vector in $R^{|T'|}$, each component of the gradient (2.2) can be computed in parallel to all others. However, the number of iterations (the critical factor of the iterative solver) must always be computed in sequence (for obvious reasons), so that the classical ELM approach can only benefit to a limited extent from parallel capabilities. For the HMM on the other hand, the situation is entirely different. The bottleneck of the HMM is the size of the state space $|X'|$, which enters the TIME complexity quadratically. In this case, however, the state space is the parallelization dimension of the Viterbi algorithm, as all states can be evaluated in parallel, but the $|T'|$ time steps of the model must be computed in sequence. Therefore, unlike for the ELM, the bottleneck of the HMM can successfully be addressed by parallelization; provided that sufficient parallel capabilities exist, the state space of an HMM can grow arbitrarily large with little impact on computational effort. The sequential time dimension in turn is, for both ELM and HMM, of $|T'| \approx 20$, considering a practical prediction horizon of 5–10 seconds.

While the HMM version of SPARC has yet to be implemented on a parallel platform (a GPU or an FPGA), the above considerations indicate that the HMM is more suited for real-time high-risk applications (such as automated driving) than the iterative optimization of an ELM.

3 Conclusion and Outlook

This paper has reviewed several key decisions in modeling and solving the SPARC concept whose early version was presented in [Zie12, RZR⁺14]. Two main points were considered of particular interest: Firstly the motivation of trading off estimated collision risks and comfort, which has been considered controversial in many instances; and secondly the decision to replace the iterative solver of the ELM with a global solver based on Hidden Markov Models, instead of improving the iterative solver heuristically. The decisions discussed here are considered the main points that set the SPARC approach apart from related approaches that have been published since then, and thus provide a reference for comparing the respective models.

Research and development on SPARC is still in progress. Current topics include validating the C^2 model for vehicle dynamics in actual test drives, not in simulations as presented in [RZW⁺14b]; collecting statistical traffic data for developing the prediction framework based on the principles presented in [RZW⁺14a]; extending the SPARC model to incorporate predictive interaction between the ego vehicle trajectory and trajectories of other traffic participants, both in cases of uncertain interaction and of coordinated cooperation between fully-automated vehicles using Car2Car communication; implementing the HMM-based solver on parallel hardware and evaluating the resulting speedup and costs; and finally integrating SPARC into a real vehicle, and validating its performance.

Bibliography

[BBF⁺08] A. Bacha, Ch. Bauman, R. Faruque, et al. Odin: Team VictorTango's entry in the DARPA Urban Challenge. *Journal of Field Robotics*, 25(8):467–492, 2008.

[CSA+09] Yi-Liang Chen, V. Sundareswaran, C. Anderson, A. Broggi, P. Grisleri, P. Porta, P. Zani, and J. Beck. TerraMax: Team Oshkosh Urban Robot. In M. Buehler, K. Iagnemma, and S. Singh, editors, *The* DARPA *Urban Challenge*, volume 56 of *Springer Tracts in Advanced Robotics*, pages 595–622. Springer Berlin Heidelberg, 2009.

[MBB+08] M. Montemerlo, J. Becker, S. Bhat, H. Dahlkamp, D. Dolgov, S. Ettinger, S. Thrun, et al. Junior: The Stanford Entry in the Urban Challenge. *Journal of Field Robotics*, 2008.

[RZR+14] M. Ruf, J.R. Ziehn, B. Rosenhahn, J. Beyerer, D. Willersinn, and H. Gotzig. Situation Prediction And Reaction Control (SPARC). In B. Färber, K. Dietmayer, K. Bengler, M. Maurer, Ch. Stiller, and H. Winner, editors, *9. Workshop Fahrerassistenzsysteme (FAS 2014)*, pages 55–66, March 2014.

[RZW+14a] M. Ruf, J.R. Ziehn, D. Willersinn, B. Rosenhahn, J. Beyerer, and H. Gotzig. A Continuous Approach to Autonomous Driving. In *Proceedings of the Conference on Vehicle and Infrastructure Safety Improvement in Adverse Conditions and Night Driving (VISION 2014)*, October 2014.

[RZW+14b] M. Ruf, J.R. Ziehn, D. Willersinn, B. Rosenhahn, J. Beyerer, and H. Gotzig. Evaluation of an Analytic Model for Car Dynamics. In *Proceedings of the IEEE International Conference on Mechatronics and Control (ICMC 2014)*, pages 2446–2451, July 2014.

[RZW+15] M. Ruf, J.R. Ziehn, D. Willersinn, B. Rosenhahn, J. Beyerer, and H. Gotzig. Global Trajectory Optimization on Multilane Roads. In *Proceedings of the IEEE 18th International Conference on Intelligent Transportation Systems (ITSC 2015)*, pages 1908–1914, September 2015.

[UAB+08] Ch. Urmson, J. Anhalt, Hong Bae, et al. Autonomous driving in urban environments: Boss and the Urban Challenge. *Journal of Field Robotics Special Issue on the 2007* DARPA *Urban Challenge, Part I*, 25(8):425–466, June 2008.

[VB10] B. Van Brunt. *The Calculus of Variations*. Springer, 2010.

[WSM09] J. Wille, F. Saust, and M. Maurer. Segmentübergreifende Bahnplanung mittels eines analytischen Optimierungsverfahrens für die autonome Fahrzeugführung auf dem Braunschweiger Stadtring. In Ch. Stiller and M. Maurer, editors, *6. Workshop Fahrerassistenzsysteme (FAS 2009)*, 2009.

[ZBDS14] J. Ziegler, P. Bender, T. Dang, and C. Stiller. Trajectory planning for Bertha – A local, continuous method. In *Intelligent Vehicles Symposium Proceedings, 2014 IEEE*, pages 450–457, June 2014.

[Zie12] J.R. Ziehn. Energy-based collision avoidance for autonomous vehicles. Master's thesis, Leibniz Universität Hannover, Germany, October 2012.

[ZRR+15] J.R. Ziehn, M. Ruf, B. Rosenhahn, D. Willersinn, J. Beyerer, and H. Gotzig. Correspondence between Variational Methods and Hidden Markov Models. In *Proceedings of the IEEE Intelligent Vehicles Symposium (IV 2015)*, pages 380–385, June 2015.

Guided Linear Dimensionality Reduction by Stochastic Gradient Descent

Matthias Richter

Vision and Fusion Laboratory
Institute for Anthropomatics
Karlsruhe Institute of Technology (KIT), Germany
matthias.richter@kit.edu

Technical Report IES-2015-05

Abstract: The aim of dimensionality reduction is to reduce the number of considered variables without removing the information needed to perform a given task. In explorative data analysis, this translates to preserving the clustering properties of the data, while in a classification setting, only class separation has to be preserved. By far the most popular tools are principal component analysis (PCA) for the former and linear discriminant analysis (LDA) for the latter. Both transform the data to a linear subspace. With PCA, the subspace is chosen so that most of the variance is preserved. However, there is no guarantee that clustering properties or even class separation are preserved too. With LDA, the data is projected to a $C - 1$ dimensional (where C denotes the number of classes) subspace so that class separation is maximized. Apart from unnecessarily restricting the number of dimensions, LDA might destroy discriminative information if its implicit assumptions (normally distributed data) are violated. In this technical report, we present a novel approach to linear dimensionality reduction. The approach is formulated as an optimization problem, which is solved using stochastic gradient descent (SGD). Like LDA, the aim is to maximize class separability. Like PCA, the dimensionality of the subspace can be specified by the user. As SGD is very sensitive to the initial conditions, we further present a method to determine suitable starting points for the gradient descent.

1 Introduction

Dimensionality reduction is the process of reducing a potentially large set of features $\mathcal{F}$ to a smaller set of features $\mathcal{F}'$ to be considered in a given machine learning or statistics problem. In an unsupervised setting, dimensionality reduction is often used for exploratory data analysis, for example to visualize the distribution of high dimensional data in human-digestible two or three dimensions. In a supervised setting, the main use is to reduce the number of parameters a learning machine has to determine. In other words: The goal of dimensionality reduction is to overcome the *curse of dimensionality* [Hug68].

A straightforward approach, *feature selection*, is to select only certain features, i.e., to choose a selection $\mathcal{F}' \subseteq \mathcal{F}$, according to some optimality criterion, e.g., related to the information content of the features in $\mathcal{F}'$ in regard to the data. More general approaches find $\mathcal{F}'$ by mapping the feature space $\mathbb{F}$ that is defined by $\mathcal{F}$ into a lower-dimensional space $\mathbb{F}'$ corresponding to $\mathcal{F}'$.

In this report, we will focus on the latter category in a supervised setting. In particular, we present a method to learn a linear mapping that approximately maximizes the distance between classes.

1.1 Related Work

Arguably the two most well known dimensionality reduction techniques are the unsupervised principal component analysis (PCA) and Fisher's supervised linear discriminant analysis (LDA). A discussion of both PCA and LDA is out of scope of this report, but can be found in numerous sources, e.g., in [DHS01].

Briefly, PCA finds a linear mapping $\mathbf{x}' = \mathbf{A}(\mathbf{x} - \overline{\mathbf{x}})$ so that the squared projection error from $\mathbf{x}$ to $\mathbf{x}'$ is minimized. The effect is that most of the data's variance in the original feature space is also represented in the reduced space $\mathbb{F}'$. Here, $\overline{\mathbf{x}}$ denotes the data's empirical mean and the columns of the matrix $\mathbf{A}$ are the eigenvectors of the data's scatter matrix (also known as the data's principal components, hence the name PCA) that correspond to the largest eigenvalues. While PCA does preserve variance, it does not necessarily preserve class separability in the projected space.

LDA, on the other hand, finds a projection so that the scatter between samples of different classes is maximized while the scatter between samples of the same class is minimized. The projection does not necessarily represent the high dimensional variation of the data well, but it does preserve information necessary to separate the classes. However, LDA makes the implicit assumption that the data of a given class are normally distributed. Coupled with the restriction that the dimensionality of $\mathbb{F}'$ is one less than the number of classes C, $\dim(\mathbb{F}') = C - 1$, this means that too much information may be discarded and the classes are not separable in $\mathbb{F}'$.

There are also nonlinear methods that project the data onto a low dimensional *manifold* embedded in $\mathbb{F}$. Examples of such methods include multidimensional scaling [Kru64], Isomap [TDSL00], local Fisher discriminant analysis [Sug07] and t-distributed stochastic neighbor embedding [VdMH08].

Dimensionality reduction also has close ties to *metric learning*, where the goal is to learn a function that realizes a distance from a given dataset. The metric is then to be used in a subsequent distance-based classifier like nearest centroid or k-nearest neighbor. Examples of metric learning methods include large margin nearest neighbor [WBS05] and information-theoric metric learning [DKJ+07]. Both methods find a metric of the form $d(\mathbf{x},\mathbf{y}) = (\mathbf{x}-\mathbf{y})^\top \mathbf{M}(\mathbf{x}-\mathbf{y})$. Although not directly applicable, metric learning can be used for dimensionality reduction if one finds a decomposition $\mathbf{M} = \mathbf{A}^\top \mathbf{A}$. This idea will be revisited in Section 2.4.

1.2 Contributions

In this technical report, we present an approach to learn a linear dimensionality reduction from a given dataset. Like LDA, the projection aims to maximize class separability. Like PCA, it allows to freely specify the dimensionality of the target space. The method is formulated as an optimization problem, which is solved using stochastic gradient descent. Furthermore, we lay a bridge between dimensionality reduction and metric learning and show how the latter can be used to aid finding solutions to the former.

2 Methods

Our method can be formalized as follows: Given a set of n-dimensional training data $\mathcal{D} = \{\mathbf{x}_1, \ldots, \mathbf{x}_N\} \subset \mathbb{R}^n$, and a partition of this set into two[1] disjoint classes $\mathcal{X}$ and $\mathcal{Y}$, the goal is to find a linear projection $\mathbf{x}' = \mathbf{A}\mathbf{x}$ into an m-dimensional space, where $m \ll n$, so that class separation is best preserved in the lower dimensional space.

[1] The method is easily extended to more than two classes, but for the sake of clarity we restrict ourselves to binary classification in this report

In other words, the goal is to find a matrix $\mathbf{A} \in \mathbb{R}^{m \times n}$ so that the squared Euclidean distance of two reduced feature vectors,

$$d_{\mathbf{A}}(\mathbf{x}, \mathbf{y}) = \|\mathbf{x}' - \mathbf{y}'\|_2^2 = \|\mathbf{A}\mathbf{x} - \mathbf{A}\mathbf{y}\|_2^2 = (\mathbf{x} - \mathbf{y})^\top \mathbf{A}^\top \mathbf{A}(\mathbf{x} - \mathbf{y}),$$

is large if $\mathbf{x}$ and $\mathbf{y}$ belong to different classes, and small otherwise. Note that this goal is very similar to that of metric learning. However, here we are explicitly interested in the dimensionality reduction so that subsequent learning algorithms do not have to be distance-based. One could use the method in [WBS05] or [DKJ+07] and decompose the matrix $\mathbf{M}$ as described in Section 2.4, but there is no guarantee that the resulting dimensionality reduction is optimal in the sense of our goal.

In this report, we instead take inspiration from LDA and find the projection matrix $\mathbf{A} = \arg\min_{\mathbf{A}} J(\mathbf{A})$ that minimizes the distance between feature vectors of the same class while simultaneously maximizing the distance between samples of different classes, measured by the unweighted ratio between intra-class and inter-class distance (like LDA),

$$J(\mathbf{A}) = \frac{S_w}{S_b} = \frac{\sum_{\mathbf{x}_u, \mathbf{x}_v \in \mathcal{X}} d_{\mathbf{A}}(\mathbf{x}_u, \mathbf{x}_v) + \sum_{\mathbf{y}_u, \mathbf{y}_v \in \mathcal{Y}} d_{\mathbf{A}}(\mathbf{y}_u, \mathbf{y}_v)}{\sum_{\mathbf{x} \in \mathcal{X}, \mathbf{y} \in \mathcal{Y}} d_{\mathbf{A}}(\mathbf{x}, \mathbf{y})}. \tag{2.1}$$

Unfortunately, a closed form solution of the above minimization problem is not readily available. Therefore, we choose to iteratively optimize eq. (2.1) instead. In particular, we employ the well known method of gradient descent to find a (local) minimum,

$$\mathbf{A}_{t+1} = \mathbf{A}_t + \Delta\mathbf{A}_t = \mathbf{A}_t - \eta_t \underbrace{\nabla_{\mathbf{A}} J(\mathbf{A}_t)}_{=:\mathbf{G}_t},$$

where $\mathbf{A}_t$ and $\Delta\mathbf{A}_t$ denote the solution candidate and update at time step t, $\mathbf{G}_t := \nabla_{\mathbf{A}} J(\mathbf{A}_t)$ denotes the gradient of the target function with respect to $\mathbf{A}$, and the hyper-parameter η_t is the learning rate at step t.

2.1 The Gradient

Key ingredient is the gradient of the target function with respect to the parameters $\mathbf{A}$. Although an approximation of the gradient using numerical differentiation (e.g., finite differences) would be possible, it would introduce a large runtime overhead as well as numerical instabilities due to discretization and round-off errors [BPR15] and should therefore be avoided. Automatic differentiation promises accurate results with negligible computational overhead [BPR15], but in our experiments we found that available implementations are still too slow for our application.

What follows is a derivation of the gradient $\nabla_{\mathbf{A}} J(\mathbf{A})$. Using the quotient rule of differentiation, the gradient expands as

$$\nabla_{\mathbf{A}} J(\mathbf{A}) = \nabla_{\mathbf{A}} \frac{S_w}{S_b} = \frac{\nabla_{\mathbf{A}} S_w \cdot S_b - S_w \cdot \nabla_{\mathbf{A}} S_b}{S_b^2}, \tag{2.2}$$

which means that we derive the gradient of S_w and S_b independently and combine the results.

As both S_w and S_b have a common structure, i.e., they are the sum of pairwise distances, we consider the gradient of the general case,

$$\begin{aligned} f(\mathbf{A}) &= \sum_{\substack{\mathbf{x}\in\mathcal{U}\\ \mathbf{y}\in\mathcal{V}}} (\mathbf{x}-\mathbf{y})^\top \mathbf{A}\mathbf{A}^\top (\mathbf{x}-\mathbf{y}) = \sum_{\substack{\mathbf{x}\in\mathcal{U}\\ \mathbf{y}\in\mathcal{V}}} \sum_{i=1}^{m} (\mathbf{x}-\mathbf{y})^\top \mathbf{a}_{:i}\mathbf{a}_{:i}^\top (\mathbf{x}-\mathbf{y}) \\ &= |\mathcal{V}| \sum_{\mathbf{x}\in\mathcal{U}} \sum_{i=1}^{m} (\mathbf{a}_{:i}^\top \mathbf{x})^2 + |\mathcal{U}| \sum_{\mathbf{y}\in\mathcal{V}} \sum_{i=1}^{m} (\mathbf{a}_{:i}^\top \mathbf{y})^2 - 2 \sum_{\substack{\mathbf{x}\in\mathcal{U}\\ \mathbf{y}\in\mathcal{V}}} \sum_{i=1}^{m} \mathbf{a}_{:i}^\top \mathbf{x}\, \mathbf{a}_{:i}^\top \mathbf{y} \end{aligned} \tag{2.3}$$

where $\mathcal{U}, \mathcal{V} \subseteq \mathcal{D}$ denote arbitrary, not necessarily disjoint subsets of the data and $\mathbf{a}_{:i}$ denotes the column-vector corresponding to the i-th column of $\mathbf{A}$. The partial derivative of eq. (2.3) with respect to a_{ik} is given as

$$\frac{\partial}{\partial a_{ik}} f(\mathbf{A}) = 2|\mathcal{V}| \sum_{\mathbf{x}\in\mathcal{U}} x_k \mathbf{a}_{:i}^\top \mathbf{x} + 2|\mathcal{U}| \sum_{\mathbf{y}\in\mathcal{U}} y_k \mathbf{a}_{:i}^\top \mathbf{y} - 2 \sum_{\substack{\mathbf{x}\in\mathcal{U}\\ \mathbf{y}\in\mathcal{V}}} \left(x_k \mathbf{a}_{:i}^\top \mathbf{y} + y_k \mathbf{a}_{:i}^\top \mathbf{x} \right). \tag{2.4}$$

To see that the above is valid, consider the function $g(\mathbf{A}) = \sum_{i=1}^{m} \left(\mathbf{a}_{:i}^\top \mathbf{x}\right)^2$. The partial derivative of this function with respect to a_{ik} is

$$\frac{\partial}{\partial a_{ik}} g(\mathbf{A}) = \frac{\partial}{\partial a_{ik}} \sum_{j=1}^{m} \left(\sum_{l=1}^{n} a_{jl} x_l \right)^2 = 2 x_k \mathbf{a}_{:i}^\top \mathbf{x},$$

which explains the first two terms of equation (2.4). Similar reasoning can be applied to derive the rightmost term. In the special case that $\mathcal{U} = \mathcal{V}$, i.e., the sum is over pairwise distances of the same set, the derivative further simplifies to

$$\frac{\partial}{\partial a_{ik}} f(\mathbf{A}) = 4(|\mathcal{U}|-1)\sum_{\mathbf{x}\in\mathcal{U}} x_k \mathbf{a}_{:i}^\top \mathbf{x} - 2\sum_{\substack{\mathbf{x},\mathbf{y}\in\mathcal{U}\\ \mathbf{x}\neq\mathbf{y}}} (x_k \mathbf{a}_{:i}^\top \mathbf{y} + y_k \mathbf{a}_{:i}^\top \mathbf{x}). \quad (2.5)$$

Putting together equations (2.4) and (2.5) yields the partial derivatives

$$\begin{aligned}\frac{\partial S_w}{\partial a_{ik}} &= 4(|\mathcal{X}|-1)\sum_{\mathbf{x}\in\mathcal{X}} x_k \mathbf{a}_{:i}^\top \mathbf{x} - 2\sum_{\substack{\mathbf{x},\mathbf{y}\in\mathcal{X}\\ \mathbf{x}\neq\mathbf{y}}} (x_k \mathbf{a}_{:i}^\top \mathbf{y} + y_k \mathbf{a}_{:i}^\top \mathbf{x}) + \\ &\quad 4(|\mathcal{Y}|-1)\sum_{\mathbf{x}\in\mathcal{Y}} x_k \mathbf{a}_{:i}^\top \mathbf{x} - 2\sum_{\substack{\mathbf{x},\mathbf{y}\in\mathcal{Y}\\ \mathbf{x}\neq\mathbf{y}}} (x_k \mathbf{a}_{:i}^\top \mathbf{y} + y_k \mathbf{a}_{:i}^\top \mathbf{x}) \quad \text{and} \quad (2.6)\\ \frac{\partial S_b}{\partial a_{ik}} &= 2|\mathcal{Y}|\sum_{\mathbf{x}\in\mathcal{X}} x_k \mathbf{a}_{:i}^\top \mathbf{x} + 2|\mathcal{X}|\sum_{\mathbf{y}\in\mathcal{Y}} y_k \mathbf{a}_{:i}^\top \mathbf{y} - 2\sum_{\substack{\mathbf{x}\in\mathcal{X}\\ \mathbf{y}\in\mathcal{Y}}}(x_k \mathbf{a}_{:i}^\top \mathbf{y} y_k \mathbf{a}_{:i}^\top \mathbf{x}). \quad (2.7)\end{aligned}$$

The partial derivatives are plugged into equation (2.2) to compute the full gradient $\nabla_{\mathbf{A}} J(\mathbf{A})$.

Note, however, that the gradient requires $(m \cdot n)$ computations – one computation for each a_{ik} – of *both* equations (2.6) and (2.7). Furthermore, the computation of both terms is quadratic in the number of training samples, which implies a very long run-time of the gradient descent, especially when large datasets are considered or a small learning rate is used.

2.2 Stochastic Gradient Descent

The field of deep learning [LBH15] faces similar, yet bigger, challenges. Here, stochastic gradient descent (SGD) has become a popular tool to speed up the learning process of deep neural networks. The main insight of SGD is that, due to the linearity of the differential operator $\nabla_{\mathbf{A}}$, the gradient of an objective function that sums over several sub-goals, $J(\mathbf{A}) = \sum_{i=1}^{N} J_i(\mathbf{A})$, can be written as

$$\nabla_{\mathbf{A}} J(\mathbf{A}) = \sum_{i=1}^{N} \nabla_{\mathbf{A}} J_i(\mathbf{A}).$$

In empirical risk minimization, one of the main pillars in machine learning, the objective function typically takes this form, where each sub-goal corresponds to minimizing the loss on one single training example.

SGD utilizes this structure by approximating the gradient with a random subsample of the training data at each step of the gradient descent,

$$\mathbf{G}_t \approx \sum_{i=1}^{K} \nabla_{\mathbf{A}} J_{\sigma_t(i)}(\mathbf{A}),$$

where $K \ll N$ is the number of samples to consider each step and σ_t is a random permutation of the set $\{1, \dots, N\}$. The intuition is that, while the individual approximations of the gradient do not point in the same direction as the true gradient, the approximation error averages out when a large number of iterations are performed. SGD requires more iterations to converge than gradient descent, but each iteration is much less computationally expensive. Thus, the overall convergence speed is generally faster, especially with large datasets or when the J_i are expensive to compute.

Unfortunately, the objective function in eq. (2.1) does not have the required structure. Both the nominator and denominator, however, do. This suggests that the general idea is applicable regardless: At each step of the gradient descent, we sample a small subset of the data, so that an equal number of samples is drawn from both $\mathcal{X}$ and $\mathcal{Y}$. The gradient $\mathbf{G}_t$ is approximated using only these samples.

2.3 AdaGrad

Stochastic gradient descent, like regular gradient descent, is very susceptible to the choice of learning rate. If the learning rate is too large, then good solutions may be missed; if it is too small, and the algorithm will converge very slowly. Ideally, the learning rate should be large in the beginning, but small when the intermediate solution is near an optimum in order not to oscillate around it.

AdaGrad [DHS11] defines a learning rate schedule that takes previous parameter updates into account. The learning rate for the (ik)-th component of the gradient is chosen as

$$\Delta a_{t,ik} = -\frac{\eta}{\sqrt{\sum_{\tau=1}^{t} g_{\tau,ik}^2}} g_{t,ik},$$

where η is a global learning rate, τ denotes the time steps before t, and $g_{\tau,ik}$ denotes the (ik)-th component of the historical gradient $\mathbf{G}_\tau$. The intuition is that larger updates will result in a smaller learning rates in the future, which effectively smoothes out extreme parameter updates due to locally steep gradients. Much like with the momentum method [RHW88] or the Newton-Raphson method, each parameter a_{ik} is associated with a different learning rate schedule, which means that the progress along each dimension of the parameter space evens out over time. A drawback is that, depending on the global learning rate, the learning rates eventually approach zero and the optimization may stop before a minimum is reached.

2.4 Initial Conditions

Another drawback of the AdaGrad schedule is that the optimization outcome is very dependent on the initial parameter estimate $\mathbf{A}_1$ [DHS11]: If the first few gradients are large (even in opposing directions), the learning rate will be slow for the remainder of the training. Additionally, in this work, the error surface defined by $J(\mathbf{A})$ is non-convex and, depending in the starting point, the gradient descent may become stuck at a shallow local minimum or saddle point.

Ideally, a good initialization would put $J(\mathbf{A})$ near a good local optimum so that the gradient descent will quickly converge towards this optimum. As was already mentioned in Section 1.1, metric learning can be used to obtain such an initialization. Given some (diagonalizable and positive semidefinite) matrix $\mathbf{M} \in \mathbb{R}^{n \times n}$, the goal is to find a decomposition $\mathbf{M} \approx \mathbf{A}^\top \mathbf{A}$ with $\mathbf{A} \in \mathbb{R}^{m \times n}$ and $m \leq n$. The matrix $\mathbf{A}$ will be used as starting point for the gradient descent.

How can such a decomposition be found? First, observe that because $\mathbf{M}$ is diagonalizable, it has the eigendecomposition

$$\mathbf{M} = \mathbf{W}\mathbf{\Lambda}\mathbf{W}^\top = \mathbf{W}\mathrm{diag}(\lambda_1, \ldots, \lambda_n)\mathbf{W}^\top,$$

where, $\mathbf{W}$ contains the eigenvectors of $\mathbf{M}$ and, by convention, the eigenvalues λ_i are sorted in descending order, $\lambda_1 \geq \lambda_2 \geq \ldots \geq \lambda_n$. Note that because $\mathbf{M}$ is positive semidefinite, all eigenvalues are non-negative, $\lambda_i \geq 0$. Similarly, $\mathbf{A}$ can be factorized using singular value decomposition,

$$\mathbf{A} = \mathbf{U}\mathbf{S}\mathbf{V}^\top = \mathbf{U}\mathrm{diag}(\sigma_1, \ldots, \sigma_m)\mathbf{V}^\top$$

where $\mathbf{S}$ contains the singular values σ_k and the orthonormal matrices $\mathbf{V}$ and $\mathbf{U}$ contain the corresponding right- and left-singular vectors of $\mathbf{A}$. Again, the singular values are sorted in descending order by convention. Combining both equations yields:

$$\begin{aligned}
\mathbf{A}^\top\mathbf{A} &= \left(\mathbf{U}\mathbf{S}\mathbf{V}^\top\right)^\top\left(\mathbf{U}\mathbf{S}\mathbf{V}^\top\right) = \mathbf{V}\mathbf{S}^\top\mathbf{S}\mathbf{V}^\top \\
&= \mathbf{V}\mathrm{diag}(\sigma_1^2, \ldots, \sigma_m^2)\mathbf{V}^\top \\
&\approx \mathbf{W}\mathrm{diag}(\lambda_1, \ldots, \lambda_n)\mathbf{W}^\top = \mathbf{M},
\end{aligned}$$

where equality holds true if $\text{rank}(\mathbf{M}) \leq m$[2]. As the λ_k are non-negative, it is possible to identify each $\sigma_k = \sqrt{\lambda_k}$ and $\mathbf{A}$ can be computed from a given $\mathbf{M}$ as

$$\mathbf{A}^\top = \mathbf{W}_{1:m,1:m}\mathbf{\Lambda}^{\frac{1}{2}}_{1:m,1:m} = \begin{pmatrix} \mathbf{e}_1^\top \\ \vdots \\ \mathbf{e}_m^\top \end{pmatrix} \text{diag}\left(\sqrt{\lambda_1}, \ldots, \sqrt{\lambda_m}\right).$$

Here, $\mathbf{W}_{1:m,1:m}$ denotes the $(m \times m)$ upper left sub-matrix of $\mathbf{W}$ (likewise $\mathbf{\Lambda}_{1:m,1:m}$). For most practical purposes, $\text{rank}(\mathbf{M}) \leq m$ does not hold. However, the *approximate* decomposition is still possible by ignoring the eigenvectors corresponding to λ_k with $k > m$. As we are only interested in a starting point for the gradient descent, an exact factorization is not necessary.

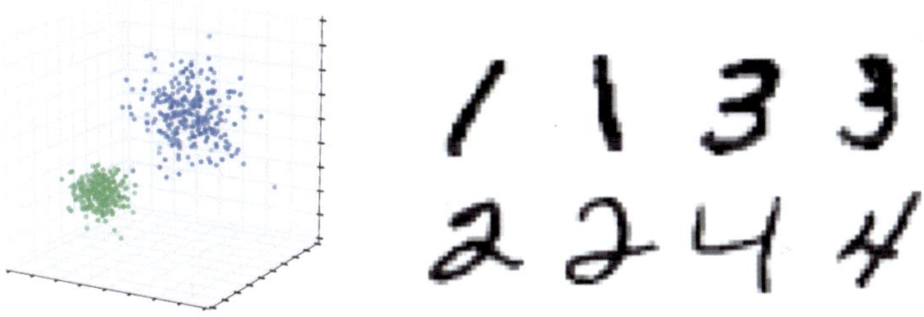

(a) Synthetic dataset (b) MNIST

Figure 3.1: Examples of the datasets used in the experiments.

3 Experiments

A prototypical implementation of our method was realized in the Julia language [BEKS14]. We implemented regular gradient descent as well as stochastic gradient descent with a fixed learning rate and with the AdaGrad learning rate schedule. In all cases, the starting point of the optimization was computed from the precision matrix of the dataset, i.e.,

[2] Since then $\lambda_k = 0$ holds for $k > m$.

$$\mathbf{A}^\top\mathbf{A} \approx \mathbf{\Sigma}^{-1} = \left(\sum_{\mathbf{x}\in\mathcal{D}}(\mathbf{x}-\overline{\mathbf{x}})(\mathbf{x}-\overline{\mathbf{x}})^\top\right)^{-1}.$$

Two experiments, one with synthetic data and one with the well known MNIST of handwritten digit dataset were carried out. In the first experiment, both $\mathcal{X}$ and $\mathcal{Y}$ were drawn from three-dimensional Gaussian distributions with different means and covariance matrices. The data was generated so that the two classes were linearly separable; hence a good dimensionality reduction should be easy to obtain. Figure 3.1(a) shows a qualitative plot of the data. The MNIST dataset contains gray value images of handwritten digits, where each image 28×28 pixels in size. In our experiments, the first class contained the digits 1 and 2, and the second class contained the digits 3 and 4. As both the digits 1 and 4 as well as 2 and 3 share similar features (e.g., vertical strokes in 1 and 4, curved lines in 2 and 3, cf. fig. 3.1(b)), the optimization is expected to produce poor results. Figure 3.1(b) show examples of the digits used in our experiment.

In both experiments, the 3- and 784-dimensional data was reduced to a 2-dimensional feature space, i.e., the projection matrix $\mathbf{A}$ had size 3×2 or 784×2 respectively.

3.1 Results

Figure 3.2 shows the value of the objective function for each iteration. With the synthetic dataset (fig. 3.2(a)), all three methods reach a local optimum very quickly. Gradient descent initially overshoots the optimum, but finds it within the next 20 iterations. SGD also overshoots, but much less so than regular gradient descent. SGD with the AdaGrad schedule finds the optimum almost immediately. With MNIST (fig. 3.2(b)), the full gradient descent did take too long to converge and is therefore missing from the plot. SGD with and without AdaGrad schedule both converge to an optimum. However the methods reach different optima, as can be seen in figure 3.3. Both methods show noisy development of the objective function that is characteristic for SGD. With AdaGrad, however, the training rate schedule suppresses larger perturbations in later iterations.

Figure 3.3 also reflects an implicit bias of our approach: it favors projections that put samples close to a linear one-dimensional manifold. This bias could be addressed by re-weighting the optimization goals, i.e., by putting more emphasis on class separation than small intra-class distance, or by introducing a non-linear projection. The latter, however, comes at the cost of a significantly more complicated gradient.

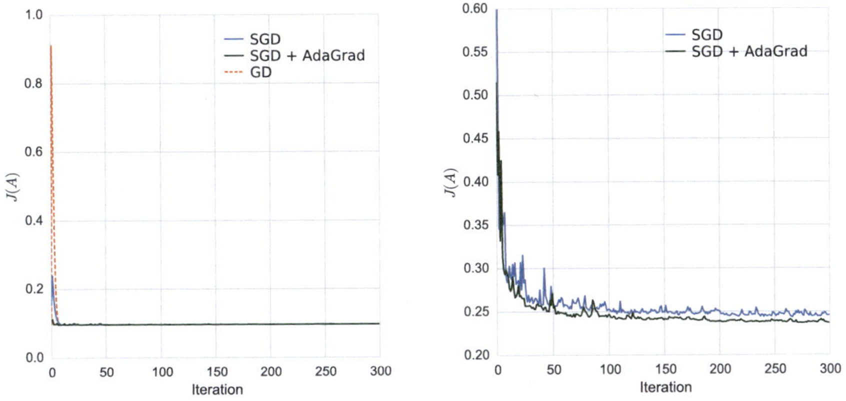

(a) Synthetic dataset (b) MNIST

Figure 3.2: Value of the objective function by iteration (best viewed in color).

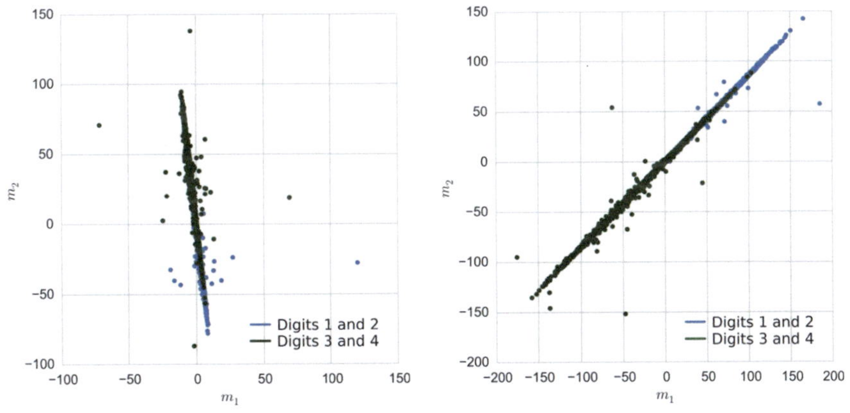

(a) SGD (b) SGD + AdaGrad

Figure 3.3: Final projection of the MNIST dataset (best viewed in color).

4 Conclusion

In this technical report, we have presented a method for linear dimensionality reduction. The method takes inspiration from both PCA and Fisher LDA and tries to minimize the pairwise distances between samples of the same class while simultaneously maximizing the distance between samples of different classes. Instead of providing a closed form solution, we chose to employ the well known gradient descent optimization algorithm. In order to speed up computation, we used stochastic gradient descent with an AdaGrad learning rate schedule.

The biggest issue with our approach is the bias to effectively reduce the features to a one-dimensional feature space. In the future, we plan to tackle this issue by re-weighting the terms of the objective function and introducing non-linearities in the projection. As this will result in a severely more complicated gradient, we will re-evaluate usage of automatic differentiation tools.

Another interesting research question concerns the use of step-wise dimensionality reduction: Instead of a direct reduction from n to m dimensions, the algorithm would first reduce the n features to $n-1$ features, then the intermediate $n-1$ features to $n-2$ features, etc., until the desired number of features is reached. The hope is that each of the intermediate reductions is easier to solve well than the full dimensionality reduction – especially if non-linearities are introduced as well.

Bibliography

[BEKS14] Jeff Bezanson, Alan Edelman, Stefan Karpinski, and Viral B Shah. Julia: A fresh approach to numerical computing. *arXiv preprint*, abs/1411.1607, 2014.

[BPR15] Atilim Gunes Baydin, Barak A. Pearlmutter, and Alexey Andreyevich Radul. Automatic differentiation in machine learning: a survey. *arXiv preprint*, abs/1502.05767, 2015.

[DHS01] Richard O. Duda, Peter E. Hart, and David G. Stork. *Pattern Classification*. Wiley-Interscience, 2 edition, November 2001.

[DHS11] John Duchi, Elad Hazan, and Yoram Singer. Adaptive subgradient methods for online learning and stochastic optimization. *The Journal of Machine Learning Research*, 12:2121–2159, 2011.

[DKJ+07] Jason V Davis, Brian Kulis, Prateek Jain, Suvrit Sra, and Inderjit S Dhillon. Information-theoretic metric learning. In *Proceedings of the 24th international conference on Machine learning*, pages 209–216. ACM, 2007.

[Hug68] G. Hughes. On the mean accuracy of statistical pattern recognizers. *IEEE Transactions on Information Theory*, 14(1):55–63, Jan 1968.

[Kru64] J. B. Kruskal. Multidimensional scaling by optimizing goodness of fit to a nonmetric hypothesis. *Psychometrika*, 29(1):1–27, 1964.

[LBH15] Yann LeCun, Yoshua Bengio, and Geoffrey Hinton. Deep learning. *Nature*, 521(7553):436–444, 2015.

[RHW88] David E Rumelhart, Geoffrey E Hinton, and Ronald J Williams. Learning representations by back-propagating errors. *Cognitive modeling*, 5(3):1, 1988.

[Sug07] Masashi Sugiyama. Dimensionality reduction of multimodal labeled data by local fisher discriminant analysis. *The Journal of Machine Learning Research*, 8:1027–1061, 2007.

[TDSL00] Joshua B Tenenbaum, Vin De Silva, and John C Langford. A global geometric framework for nonlinear dimensionality reduction. *science*, 290(5500):2319–2323, 2000.

[VdMH08] Laurens Van der Maaten and Geoffrey Hinton. Visualizing data using t-sne. *Journal of Machine Learning Research*, 9(2579-2605):85, 2008.

[WBS05] Kilian Q Weinberger, John Blitzer, and Lawrence K Saul. Distance metric learning for large margin nearest neighbor classification. In *Advances in neural information processing systems*, pages 1473–1480, 2005.

Fast Polarization State Detection by Division-of-Amplitude in a Simple Configuration Setup

Christian Negara

Fraunhofer Institute of Optronics,
System Technologies and Image Exploitation IOSB
Fraunhoferstr. 1, 76131 Karlsruhe, Germany
christian.negara@iosb.fraunhofer.de

Technical Report IES-2015-06

Abstract: A new measurement system for imaging ellipsometry has been developed with the ability of taking fast measurements on planar and even highly curved surfaces. This is achieved by a special laser scanner containing four photodetectors to measure the state of polarization with a sampling rate in the megahertz range. Up to now only three of four Stokes parameters can be measured simultaneously. In this work some modifications to the actual detector are proposed which provide the opportunity to measure the whole Stokes parameter. In contrast to the previous work on the division-of-amplitude photopolarimeter (DOAP) using a special optical beam splitter, the polarization state detector presented here uses only standard optical components while keeping the adjustment effort low.

1 Introduction

Ellipsometry is a sensitive technique for thickness measurement of thin films. Most measuring systems based on ellipsometry require a precise adjustment of the input and output heads down to 0.1° to satisfy the reflection condition. Therefore, measurements are performed only at nearly flat surfaces. Recently, a new measurement system for ellipsometry has been developed at Fraunhofer IOSB, which circumvents this restriction by using a retroreflector as shown in Figure 1.1. The differences and similarities to an usual ellipsometer are explained in [Neg15, NII14], especially the change of the ellipsometric parameters Ψ, Δ and the number of occuring ambiguities.

A precise measurement of the thickness or other material properties requires a precise measurement of the state of polarization i.e. Stokes parameter of the reflected light by the polarization state detector (PSD). It can be shown that the four elements of the Stokes parameter can be measured by four measurements. One possibility for the realization of the PSD is the division-of-amplitude photopolarimeter (DOAP) [Azz82]. One element of this PSD is a special beam splitter. There are optimality constraints on the optical properties of the beam splitter [AD03] to maximize the sensitivity of the PSD. In [YSZL14] a beam splitter was realized and validated consisting of 46 dielectric layers whose optical properties are near the theoretical optimum. One drawback of this multilayer beam splitter is the high production cost which increases the cost for the PSD. In [AS05] a single-layer beam splitter was proposed which also has good polarization properties. A drawback of both beam splitters is the need for a special single- or multilayer coating. The production costs for optical coatings are only low if several beam splitters are coated simultaneously and hence several PSDs are produced.

To build up a PSD in a prototypical manner for measuring the full Stokes parameter, an alternative configuration is proposed consisting only of standard and cheap optical components like quarter-wave plates and standard beam splitters while still reaching 91% of the theoretical optimal value. Furthermore, a beam splitter is proposed which has no special coating despite of the antireflective coating on the front- and backside. The optical polarization properties of this beam splitter in combination with four quarter-wave plates would be also near the optimum.

1.1 Design of an Ellipsometer with a Retroreflector

In contrast to the standard ellipsometry configuration, the usage of a retroreflector circumvents the need for a separate detector head to measure the state of polarization. Instead, the excitation head for the light source and the detector head with the PSD are combined together into a transceiver. The outgoing and ingoing beams are made collinear by a nonpolarized beam splitter. In Figure 1.2 the optical path inside the transceiver is depicted. By a fast rotating polygon mirror in the deflection unit a laser line is obtained from a laser beam. This allows the appliance of the laser scanner for imaging ellipsometry. The line frequency of the prototype is 1 kHz and the line width 12 cm. The pixel frequency rate is approximately 2 MHz. The input beam is further split up by beam splitters so that four intensity measurements are obtained by four photomultipliers for the detection of the state of polarization. The advantage of using photomultipliers as photodetectors is a high sampling rate at low intensities. This is needed because the light is reflected twice off the sample surface. If the sample is illuminated by nonpolarized light and R is the reflectance of the sample, R^2 is the reflectance measured in the configuration with a retroreflector. The intensity is furthermore lowered because a non-ideal retroreflector reflects an incident light beam as a light cone.

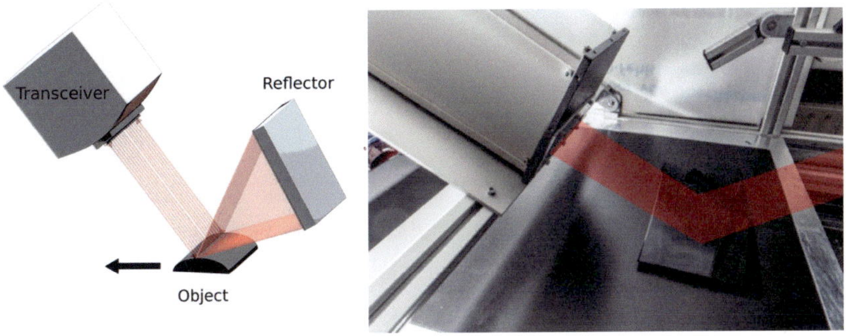

(a) (b)

Figure 1.1: Scheme of the beam path with retroreflection (a) and an image of the ellipsometry scanner (b).

1.2 Stokes Parameter and Mueller Calculus

One convenient way describing the state of polarization for totally, as well as partly polarized light, is by a four-dimensional Stokes parameter $\boldsymbol{S} \in \mathbb{R}^4$. The Stokes parameter of a light ray is referenced to a fixed right-handed coordinate system (x, y, z) while the z-axis points to the observer. The conventions about the coordinate systems and transformations used in this paper follow the Nebraska ellipsometry conventions [HMS80]. The definition of the Stokes parameter $\boldsymbol{S}$ is [Fuj07]:

$$\boldsymbol{S} = \begin{pmatrix} S_0 \\ S_1 \\ S_2 \\ S_3 \end{pmatrix} = \begin{pmatrix} I_{0^\circ} + I_{90^\circ} \\ I_{0^\circ} - I_{90^\circ} \\ I_{45^\circ} - I_{-45^\circ} \\ I_R - I_L \end{pmatrix}$$

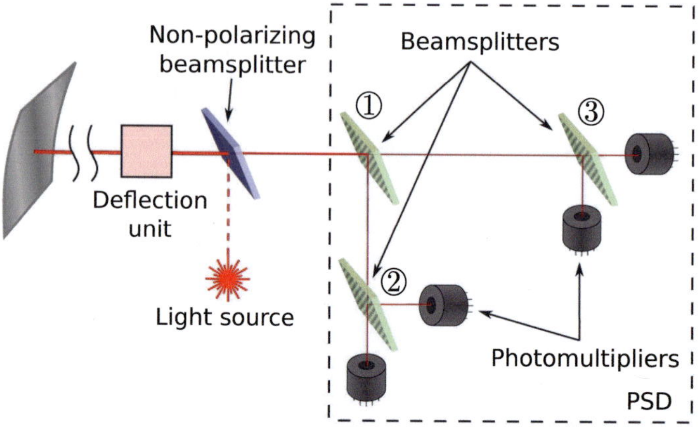

Figure 1.2: Design of the PSD inside the transceiver.

whereas $I_{0^\circ}, I_{90^\circ}, I_{45^\circ}, I_{-45^\circ}$ are the measured light intensities after the light ray passes rotated linear polarizers at $0^\circ, 45^\circ, 90^\circ, -45^\circ$ and I_R, I_L are the measured intensities after it passes left and right circular polarizers. Therefore, the definition already gives one possibility to measure the Stokes parameter, although six measurements would be needed. Orthogonal polarization states are coupled by the following identity which gives the intensity S_0 of the light:

$$S_0 = I_{0^\circ} + I_{90^\circ} = I_{45^\circ} + I_{-45^\circ} = I_L + I_R$$

Furthermore the following inequality holds:

$$S_1^2 + S_2^2 + S_3^2 \leq S_0^2 \,. \tag{1.1}$$

From the Stokes parameter the degree of polarization P can be defined as:

$$P = \frac{\sqrt{S_1^2 + S_2^2 + S_3^2}}{S_0} \,.$$

For completely polarized light ($P = 1$) the less-or-equal sign in Equation (1.1) is replaced by the equal sign.

The transformation of the Stokes parameter of a light ray when it passes an optical element can be described by the so-called Mueller matrix $\mathbf{M} \in \mathbb{R}^{4\times4}$. The Stokes parameter $\boldsymbol{S}^{in}$ of a light ray successively passing through several optical components with the Mueller matrices $\mathbf{M}_1, \ldots, \mathbf{M}_n$ is transformed into the

Stokes parameter

$$\boldsymbol{S}^{out} = \underbrace{\mathbf{M}_n \cdot \mathbf{M}_{n-1} \cdot \ldots \cdot \mathbf{M}_1}_{=:\mathbf{M}} \cdot \boldsymbol{S}^{in}$$

whereas $\boldsymbol{S}^{out}$ is the Stokes parameter of the outgoing light ray. If the light ray hits a photodetector after it passes several optical elements only the intensity part S_0^{out} of $\boldsymbol{S}^{out}$ is measured, because most photodetectors are insensitive to the state of polarization. The measured intensity S_0^{out} can be computed by:

$$S_0^{out} = [\mathbf{M}]_{(1,1..4)} \cdot \boldsymbol{S}^{in}$$

while $[\mathbf{M}]_{(1,1..4)}$ is the first row of $\mathbf{M}$.

If the Mueller matrix $\mathbf{M}$ of an optical element is given which changes the Stokes parameter of an incoming light ray, the Mueller matrix of an optical element rotated around the z-axis (directional vector of the light ray) can also be computed. For an optical element with the Mueller matrix $\mathbf{M}$ given in (x', y') coordinates which is rotated by an angle α relative to the x-axis as shown in Figure 1.3 the Mueller matrix $\mathbf{M}_R(\mathbf{M}, \alpha)$ of the rotated optical component given in (x, y) coordinates becomes:

$$\mathbf{M}_R(\mathbf{M}, \alpha) = \mathbf{R}(-\alpha) \cdot \mathbf{M} \cdot \mathbf{R}(\alpha) \tag{1.2}$$

where

$$\mathbf{R}(\alpha) = \begin{pmatrix} 1 & 0 & 0 & 0 \\ 0 & \cos 2\alpha & \sin 2\alpha & 0 \\ 0 & -\sin 2\alpha & \cos 2\alpha & 0 \\ 0 & 0 & 0 & 1 \end{pmatrix} . \tag{1.3}$$

Equation (1.2) results from two transformations. First the Stokes parameter of the emitted light ray in (x, y) coordinates is transformed to (x', y') coordinates by multiplying the Stokes parameter with $\mathbf{R}(\alpha)$. The Stokes parameter in (x', y') coordinates can then be multiplied by the Mueller matrix $\mathbf{M}$ of the rotated optical element which is defined in (x', y') coordinates. To compute the Stokes parameter according to the primary coordinate system (x, y) a second transformation is applied by multiplying the Stokes parameter with $\mathbf{R}(-\alpha)$ which changes the (x', y') coordinates back to (x, y) coordinates. It should be noted that the same Mueller matrix is obtained if an optical element is rotated by $180°$ degrees (see Equation (1.3)) because the total phase of a light wave is disregarded in Mueller calculus.

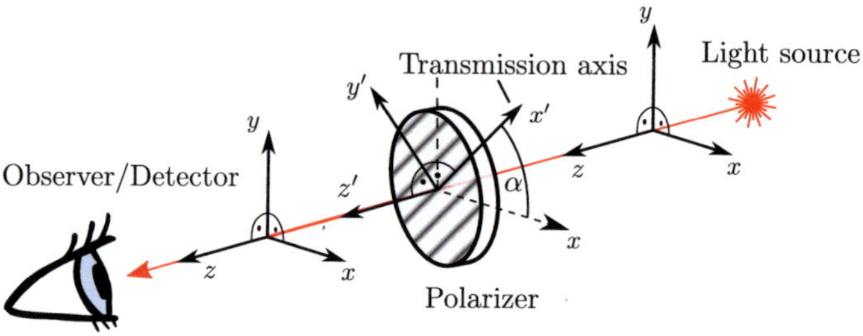

Figure 1.3: Transformation of the coordinate system for a rotated polarizer.

Two important ellipsometry parameters that are measured by ellipsometers are the ellipsometric parameters Ψ and Δ which can be combined to a complex value $\underline{\rho}$. Ψ describes the change in the amplitude quotient and Δ the change in the phase difference of two orthogonal linearly polarized waves. Because the coordinate system of the ellipsometer is adjusted according to the plane of incidence (see Figure 1.4), the two linearly polarized waves correspond to the s- and p-polarization. The ellipsometric parameters Ψ, Δ are then related to the complex reflection coefficients $\underline{r}^p, \underline{r}^s$ of the sample by the fundamental equation of ellipsometry [TM99]:

$$\underline{\rho}_r := \tan \Psi_r \mathrm{e}^{i\Delta_r} = \frac{\underline{r}^p}{\underline{r}^s}.$$

where the subscript r denotes that the measurements are made in reflection. Ellipsometry can also be applied in transmission and in this case we get:

$$\underline{\rho}_t := \tan \Psi_t \mathrm{e}^{i\Delta_t} = \frac{\underline{t}^p}{\underline{t}^s}.$$

where the variables $\underline{t}^p, \underline{t}^s$ are the complex transmission coefficients.

From the reflection coefficients $\underline{r}^p, \underline{r}^s$ describing the ratio of amplitudes of the electric fields, the reflectance R_s^2, R_p^2 describing the ratio of intensities can be computed by $R_s = |\underline{r}^s|^2, R_p = |\underline{r}^p|^2$. An averaged value of the reflectance can further be defined as $R = (R_s + R_p)/2$ which corresponds to the overall intensity ratio for nonpolarized or circularly polarized incident light. In the nonabsorbing case (e.g. nonabsorbing beam splitters) the reflectance R and transmittance T satisfy the following condition $R + T = 1$.

When measuring a sample in reflection, which is isotropic and nondepolarizing, the corresponding Mueller matrix $\mathbf{M}_S(\Psi_r, \Delta_r, R)$ for the ellipsometric parameters Ψ_r, Δ_r and the reflectance R is:

$$\mathbf{M}_S(\Psi_r,\Delta_r,R) = R\begin{pmatrix} 1 & -\cos 2\Psi_r & 0 & 0 \\ -\cos 2\Psi_r & 1 & 0 & 0 \\ 0 & 0 & \sin 2\Psi_r \cos\Delta_r & \sin 2\Psi_r \sin\Delta_r \\ 0 & 0 & -\sin 2\Psi_r \sin\Delta_r & \sin 2\Psi_r \cos\Delta_r \end{pmatrix}.$$

The sample could also be a beam splitter and Ψ_r, Δ_r, R the parameters for the reflected ray. Analogous, a sample (e.g. a beam splitter) could also be measured in transmission and if Ψ_t, Δ_t are the ellipsometric parameters and T the transmittance of the transmitted ray the Mueller matrix becomes $\mathbf{M}_S(\Psi_t, \Delta_t, T)$.

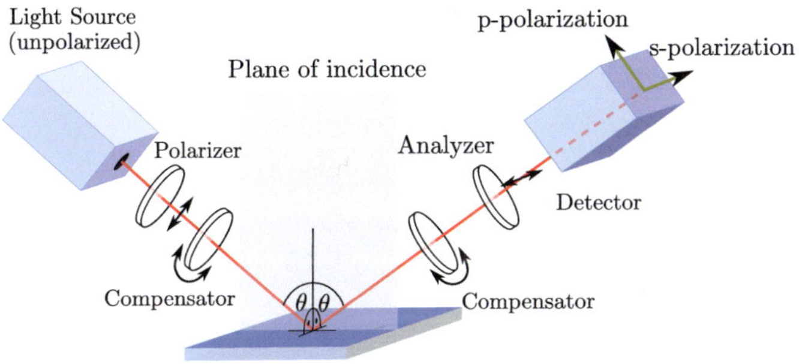

Figure 1.4: Conventional configuration of an ellipsometer.

2 Previous Work

2.1 Optical Properties of the Actual Detector

The actual design of the detector splits the incoming light ray into four rays through nonpolarizing and polarizing beam splitters (see Figure 1.2). First the incoming light ray is split up by a nonpolarizing beam splitter ① with $R = T = 0.5$ thus obtaining two rays with equal polarization and half of the intensity which corresponds to the Mueller matrix

$$\mathbf{M}_\mathrm{N} = \frac{1}{2}\begin{pmatrix} 1 & 0 & 0 & 0 \\ 0 & 1 & 0 & 0 \\ 0 & 0 & 1 & 0 \\ 0 & 0 & 0 & 1 \end{pmatrix}$$

One of the two rays is further split up by a polarizing beam splitter ② rotated at 0°. The other by a polarizing beam splitter ③ rotated at 45°. The polarizing beam splitters split up the state of polarization of the incoming ray in a p-polarized transmitted and s-polarized reflected ray (see Figure 2.1).

The Mueller matrix $\mathbf{M}_{\text{Pol,t}}$ for the transmitted ray of an ideal polarizing beam splitter with a transmittance of 100% for the p-polarization ($T_p = 1$) and 0% for the s-polarization ($T_s = 0$) is

$$\mathbf{M}_{\text{Pol,t}} = \frac{1}{2} \begin{pmatrix} 1 & 1 & 0 & 0 \\ 1 & 1 & 0 & 0 \\ 0 & 0 & 0 & 0 \\ 0 & 0 & 0 & 0 \end{pmatrix}$$

whereas the Mueller matrix $\mathbf{M}_{\text{Pol,r}}$ for the reflected ray with reflectance of $R_p = 0$ and $R_s = 1$ is

$$\mathbf{M}_{\text{Pol,r}} = \frac{1}{2} \begin{pmatrix} 1 & -1 & 0 & 0 \\ -1 & 1 & 0 & 0 \\ 0 & 0 & 0 & 0 \\ 0 & 0 & 0 & 0 \end{pmatrix} .$$

$\mathbf{M}_{\text{Pol,t}}$ is the Mueller matrix of a polarizer rotated at $0°$ because the x-axis corresponds to the p-polarization and the y-axis to the s-polarization according to convention. Therefore, $\mathbf{M}_{\text{Pol,r}}$ is the Mueller matrix of a polarizer rotated at $90°$ according to Equation (1.3). More generally $\mathbf{M}_{\text{Pol},\alpha}$ will denote the Mueller matrix of a polarizer rotated at an angle α. For the polarizing beam splitter rotated at $45°$ the Mueller matrix for the transmitted ray is

$$\mathbf{M}_{\text{Pol},45°} = \frac{1}{2} \begin{pmatrix} 1 & 0 & -1 & 0 \\ 0 & 0 & 0 & 0 \\ -1 & 0 & 1 & 0 \\ 0 & 0 & 0 & 0 \end{pmatrix}$$

and for the reflected ray

$$\mathbf{M}_{\text{Pol},-45°} = \frac{1}{2} \begin{pmatrix} 1 & 0 & 1 & 0 \\ 0 & 0 & 0 & 0 \\ 1 & 0 & 1 & 0 \\ 0 & 0 & 0 & 0 \end{pmatrix} .$$

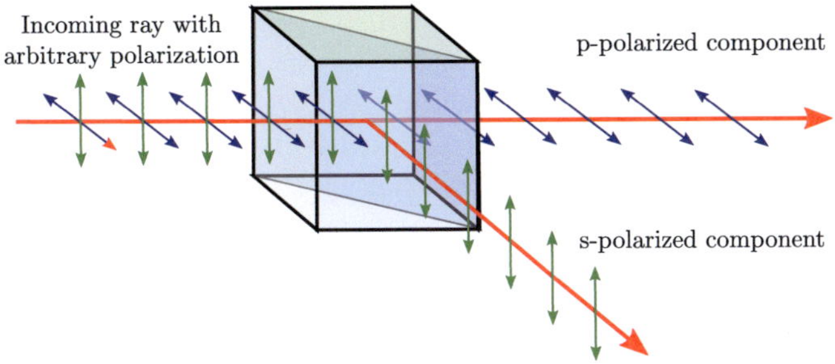

Figure 2.1: Transmission and reflection at a polarizing beam splitter.

A special mounting has been constructed to fix the photomultipliers and the beam splitter at an angle of rotation of $45°$. A special mounting is needed because the plane of incidence changes from the first to the second beam splitter (rotated at $45°$).

The intensities $I_1, \ldots, I_4$ measured by the photodetectors, which can be combined to a vector $\boldsymbol{I}$, can be computed from the Stokes parameter $\boldsymbol{S}^{in}$ by the so-called instrument matrix $\mathbf{A} \in \mathbb{R}^{4\times4}$

$$\boldsymbol{I} = \mathbf{A} \cdot \boldsymbol{S}^{in} \ .$$

The instrument matrix of the actual design of the detector is

$$\mathbf{A}_{\text{Act}} = \begin{pmatrix} [\mathbf{M}_N \cdot \mathbf{M}_{\text{Pol},0°}]_{(1,1..4)} \\ [\mathbf{M}_N \cdot \mathbf{M}_{\text{Pol},90°}]_{(1,1..4)} \\ [\mathbf{M}_N \cdot \mathbf{M}_{\text{Pol},45°}]_{(1,1..4)} \\ [\mathbf{M}_N \cdot \mathbf{M}_{\text{Pol},-45°}]_{(1,1..4)} \end{pmatrix} = \begin{pmatrix} 1 & 1 & 0 & 0 \\ 1 & -1 & 0 & 0 \\ 1 & 0 & -1 & 0 \\ 1 & 0 & 1 & 0 \end{pmatrix} .$$

As can be seen $\mathbf{A}_{\text{Act}}$ is not invertible. Therefore it is not possible to compute all four elements of the Stokes parameter $\boldsymbol{S}^{out}$ from the measurements. It is neither possible to compute the degree of polarization to study samples with depolarization nor to compute Δ in the maximum possible range from $[0°, 180°]$ – just in the range from $[0°, 90°]$. The full interval $[0°, 360°]$ of Δ which can be measured with conventional ellipsometers cannot be determined in the configuration with a retroreflector [Neg15, NH14].

2.2 Division-of-Amplitude Photopolarimeter

A very similar design of the polarization state detector to the one presented in Section 2.1 has been proposed in [Azz82] as the division of amplitude photopolarimeter. In contrast to the nonpolarized beam splitter ① used in the previous section, a special beam splitter is used which is optimal regarding the optimality criterion. As the optimality criterion the absolute value of the determinant of the instrument matrix [AD03] has been chosen, which has to be maximized. Despite of the nonpolarizing beam splitter the design of the DOAP also differs from the one presented in Section 2.1 by the polarizing beam splitters ② and ③ which are both rotated at $45°$[1]. The effect of the beam splitter ① on the state of polarization can be characterized by (Ψ_r, Δ_r, R) for the reflected ray and (Ψ_t, Δ_t, T) for the transmitted ray which results in the Mueller matrices $\mathbf{M}_S(\Psi_r, \Delta_r, R)$ and $\mathbf{M}_S(\Psi_t, \Delta_t, T)$, respectively. For this configuration the instrument matrix becomes

$$\mathbf{A}_{\text{DOAP}} = \begin{pmatrix} [\mathbf{M}_{\text{Pol},45°} \cdot \mathbf{M}_S(\Psi_r, \Delta_r, R)]_{(1,1..4)} \\ [\mathbf{M}_{\text{Pol},-45°} \cdot \mathbf{M}_S(\Psi_r, \Delta_r, R)]_{(1,1..4)} \\ [\mathbf{M}_{\text{Pol},45°} \cdot \mathbf{M}_S(\Psi_t, \Delta_t, T)]_{(1,1..4)} \\ [\mathbf{M}_{\text{Pol},-45°} \cdot \mathbf{M}_S(\Psi_t, \Delta_t, T)]_{(1,1..4)} \end{pmatrix}$$

and the determinant

$$\det \mathbf{A}_{\text{DOAP}} = \frac{1}{4} R^2 T^2 (\cos 2\Psi_r - \cos 2\Psi_t) \sin 2\Psi_r \sin 2\Psi_t \sin(\Delta_r - \Delta_t)\,. \quad (2.1)$$

For nonpolarizing beam splitters the equality $\Psi_r = \Psi_t = 45°$ holds and in that case the determinant becomes zero independent of Δ_r, Δ_t and R, T. This is also true for the case where the beam splitters ② and ③ are rotated by an arbitrary angle. Therefore an unpolarizing beam splitter cannot be used to measure all elements of the Stokes parameter. It should also be noted that the determinant becomes zero independent of the optical properties of the beam splitter when the beam splitters ② and ③ are rotated by $0°$ instead of $45°$. The optimal values which maximizes $|\det \mathbf{A}_{\text{DOAP}}|$ are [AD03]

$$\begin{aligned} \Delta_r - \Delta_t &= \pm\pi/2, \\ R = T &= 0.5, \\ \Psi_r &= \frac{1}{2} \arccos(\pm 1/\sqrt{3}) \\ \Psi_t &= \pi/2 - \Psi_r \end{aligned} \quad (2.2)$$

[1] Instead of polarizing beam splitters Wollaston prisms are used, but the Mueller matrices are equal.

and $\det_{\max}$ is defined by[2] $\det_{\max} := \max|\det \mathbf{A}_{\text{DOAP}}| = \sqrt{3}/144$. The equation $\Psi_t = \pi/2 - \Psi_r$ is always true if $R = T = 0.5$ i.e. the beam splitter is non-absorbing and the intensities in both optical paths are split equally. For this case Equation (2.1) simplifies to:

$$\det \mathbf{A}_{\text{DOAP}} = \frac{1}{64} \sin 2\Psi_r \sin 4\Psi_r \sin(\Delta_r - \Delta_t) \,. \tag{2.3}$$

In the rest of the paper the focus will rely on beam splitters with $R = T = 0.5$.

To measure how close a special design of the PSD reaches the optimal value, the normalized determinant can be defined as follows:

$$|\det \mathbf{A}|_{\text{norm}} := \frac{|\det \mathbf{A}|}{\det_{\max}} \tag{2.4}$$

A special beam splitter prism with a single-layer coating was proposed in [AS05] which has a normalized determinant of 0.85 at $633\ \text{nm}$. The angle of incidence is 77° so a special alignment as well as a special geometry of the beam splitter is needed.

3 An Alternative Design of the PSD

In this work another configuration of the PSD is proposed where quater-wave plates are mounted at the transmitted as well as the reflected optical path of the beam splitter ①. Furthermore, the polarizing beam splitters ② and ③ are both rotated at 0°. The Mueller matrix of an ideal quarter-wave plate (with antireflective coating) is

$$\mathbf{M}_{\frac{\lambda}{4}} - \begin{pmatrix} 1 & 0 & 0 & 0 \\ 0 & 1 & 0 & 0 \\ 0 & 0 & 0 & 1 \\ 0 & 0 & -1 & 0 \end{pmatrix}$$

and the Mueller matrix of a quarter-wave plate rotated by an angle α will be denoted as $\mathbf{M}_{\frac{\lambda}{4},\alpha}$.

[2] The factor $1/4$ is disregarded in the referenced literature

When one quarter-wave plate is mounted at each optical path and rotated by angles α_r and α_t, respectively, the instrument matrix becomes

$$\mathbf{A}_{\frac{\lambda}{4}} = \begin{pmatrix} \left[\mathbf{M}_{\mathrm{Pol},0^\circ} \cdot \mathbf{M}_{\frac{\lambda}{4},\alpha_r} \cdot \mathbf{M}_S(\Psi_r, \Delta_r, R)\right]_{(1,1..4)} \\ \left[\mathbf{M}_{\mathrm{Pol},90^\circ} \cdot \mathbf{M}_{\frac{\lambda}{4},\alpha_r} \cdot \mathbf{M}_S(\Psi_r, \Delta_r, R)\right]_{(1,1..4)} \\ \left[\mathbf{M}_{\mathrm{Pol},0^\circ} \cdot \mathbf{M}_{\frac{\lambda}{4},\alpha_t} \cdot \mathbf{M}_S(\Psi_t, \Delta_t, T)\right]_{(1,1..4)} \\ \left[\mathbf{M}_{\mathrm{Pol},90^\circ} \cdot \mathbf{M}_{\frac{\lambda}{4},\alpha_t} \cdot \mathbf{M}_S(\Psi_t, \Delta_t, T)\right]_{(1,1..4)} \end{pmatrix}$$

whereas $T = 1 - R$ and $\Psi_t = \pi/2 - \Psi_r$. If $\Delta_r = \pi$ and $\Delta_t = 0$ the determinant of the Mueller matrix $\mathbf{A}_{\frac{\lambda}{4}}$ becomes:

$$\det \mathbf{A}_{\frac{\lambda}{4}} = \frac{1}{64} \sin 2\Psi_r \sin 4\Psi_r \underbrace{\sin 2\alpha_r \sin 2\alpha_t (\cos 2\alpha_t - \cos 2\alpha_r)}_{=:f(\alpha_r,\alpha_t)} . \quad (3.1)$$

Comparing Equation (3.1) with (2.1) reveals that optimal solutions for α_r, α_t can be found in Equation (2.2) e.g. $\alpha_r = \frac{1}{2}\arccos(1/\sqrt{3}) \approx 27.37°$ and $\alpha_t = \pi/2 - \alpha_r \approx 62.63°$. The maximum value of $|f(\alpha_r, \alpha_t)|$ is approximately 0.77 and this is also the maximum of $|\det \mathbf{A}_{\frac{\lambda}{4}}|_{\mathrm{norm}}$ which results from Equation (2.3).

There are two differences of the DOAP in Section 2.2 and the DOAP with quarter-wave plates presented here. First, the polarizing beam splitters ② and ③ are not tilted, hence all light rays remain in one single plane of incidence, which simplifies the mounting of the photodetectors. Second, $\Delta_r = \pi$ and $\Delta_t = 0$, which is more natural for an uncoated surface illuminated by light at an angle of incidence of $45°$, because $45°$ is below the brewster angle of glasses ($> 50°$). In both cases the instrument matrix $\mathbf{A}_{\mathrm{DOAP}}$ in the previous section is singular.

To get better results for the normalized determinant from Equation (2.4) one possibility is to add two more quarter-wave plates as shown in Figure 3.1. The angles of rotation of the second quarter-wave plates in comparison to the first quarter-wave plates differ by α_Δ. In this case it is possible to find angles of rotation $(\alpha_r, \alpha_t, \alpha_\Delta)$ for which the normalized determinant is equal to 1. The instrument matrix $\mathbf{A}'_{\frac{\lambda}{4}}$ with four quarter-wave plates is

$$\mathbf{A}'_{\frac{\lambda}{4}} = \begin{pmatrix} \left[\mathbf{M}_{\text{Pol},0^\circ} \cdot \mathbf{M}_{\frac{\lambda}{4},\alpha_r+\alpha_\Delta} \cdot \mathbf{M}_{\frac{\lambda}{4},\alpha_r} \cdot \mathbf{M}_S(\Psi_r,\pi,R)\right]_{(1,1..4)} \\ \left[\mathbf{M}_{\text{Pol},90^\circ} \cdot \mathbf{M}_{\frac{\lambda}{4},\alpha_r+\alpha_\Delta} \cdot \mathbf{M}_{\frac{\lambda}{4},\alpha_r} \cdot \mathbf{M}_S(\Psi_r,\pi,R)\right]_{(1,1..4)} \\ \left[\mathbf{M}_{\text{Pol},0^\circ} \cdot \mathbf{M}_{\frac{\lambda}{4},\alpha_t+\alpha_\Delta} \cdot \mathbf{M}_{\frac{\lambda}{4},\alpha_t} \cdot \mathbf{M}_S(\Psi_t,0,T)\right]_{(1,1..4)} \\ \left[\mathbf{M}_{\text{Pol},90^\circ} \cdot \mathbf{M}_{\frac{\lambda}{4},\alpha_t+\alpha_\Delta} \cdot \mathbf{M}_{\frac{\lambda}{4},\alpha_t} \cdot \mathbf{M}_S(\Psi_t,0,T)\right]_{(1,1..4)} \end{pmatrix}$$

whereas the determinant of $\mathbf{A}'_{\frac{\lambda}{4}}$ becomes

$$\det \mathbf{A}'_{\frac{\lambda}{4}} = \frac{1}{64} \sin 2\Psi_r \sin 4\Psi_r f'(\alpha_r, \alpha_t, \alpha_\Delta) .$$

while f' is a function of the angles of rotation $(\alpha_r, \alpha_t, \alpha_\Delta)$ and is not presented here due to its length. In contrast to f the maximum value of $|f'(\alpha_r, \alpha_t, \alpha_\Delta)|$ is 1 and hence the PSD is optimal because its normalized determinant is 1. Instead of an analytical solution optimal values for the angles of rotation can be simply found by nonlinear optimization. This was tested in *Mathematica* where optimal values were always found. For example the following solution

$$\begin{aligned} \Psi_r &= 27.4^\circ \\ \alpha_r &= 0^\circ \\ \alpha_t &= 45^\circ \\ \alpha_\Delta &= 45^\circ \end{aligned}$$

would result in a normalized determinant of $\approx 1 - 10^{-5}$.

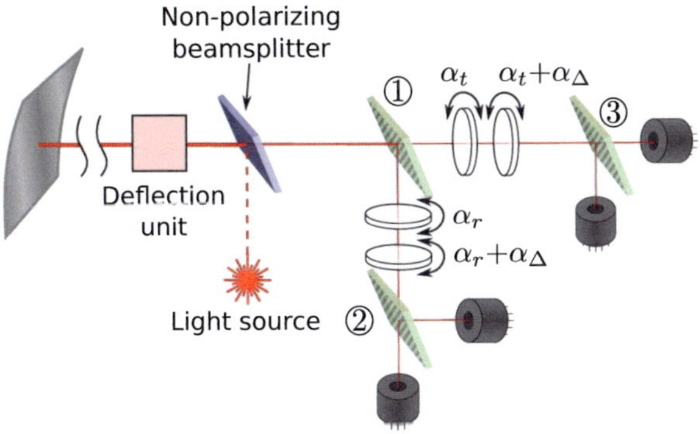

Figure 3.1: Design of the PSD with quarter-wave plates.

When the phase differences Δ_r and Δ_t are not 0 or π as defined above, it is also possible to find an optimal configuration for the angles of rotation of the quarter-wave plates. In this case $(\alpha_r, \alpha_t, \alpha_{\Delta_t}) \neq (0°, 45°, 45°)$ but the optimal values can be found with the same nonlinear optimization algorithm. Simulations with random values for Δ_r and Δ_t show that it is always possible to find a configuration for which the normalized determinant of the instrument matrix becomes 1 as long as Ψ_r is optimal as defined in Equation (2.2). For many commercially available beam splitters Ψ_r and Ψ_t are specified but Δ_r and Δ_t are not. In this case they could be measured with an ellipsometer and afterwards $(\alpha_r, \alpha_t, \alpha_\Delta)$ could be adjusted according to the measured values of Δ_r and Δ_t to get optimal results to maximize the normalized determinant.

4 Conclusion

In contrast to previous designs of the PSD all light rays are traversing a single plane of incidence and the angles of the refracted and reflected rays are always $90°$ which makes it easy to build up and test the PSD on a microbench in a prototypical manner. No restriction on Δ_r and Δ_t is needed anymore, which makes it more easy to find cheap beam splitters with optical properties near the optimum. A standard beam splitter cube from *Edmund Optics* with $R_p = 0.88$ and $R_s = 0.27$ at $\lambda = 633$ nm costs $< 200\$$ and would still reach 91% of the optimal value of the determinant of the instrument matrix. The cost for the optical components of the PSD would be therefore much cheaper than specially coated beam splitters with single or multi-layers which could reach several thousands of dollars. This applies in particular to single pieces such as prototypes while the cost for the production of several beam splitters with a special multilayer coating would be lower.

What is even more important than the saving of costs is the wavelength dependency of Ψ, Δ especially for multilayer coatings. For beam splitters with multilayer coatings it was shown in previous work that the normalized determinant decreases if the wavelength differs from the design wavelength. It is probably very difficult to satisfy the optimality conditions on Ψ_r, Δ_r, R and Ψ_t, Δ_t, T over a broad wavelength range in one multilayer coating because usually they are chosen to obtain only one given wavelength-dependent function e.g. $R(\lambda)$. By decoupling the optical properties of the PSD from a single (multilayer) coating into three optical elements, it is easier to get near-optimal results over a broad wavelength range. Furthermore, if the wavelength is tuned over time the ratardance at the transmitted and refracted ray could also be tuned to get optimal results by replacing the quarter-wave plates by photoelectric modulators (PEM).

The only drawback of the presented DOAP is the need for additional quarter-wave plates but in contrast to special beam splitters they are manufactured in bulk and are therefore cheap. They are also available with special holders which allows the fixation at given angles of rotation.

Bibliography

[AD03] Azzam, R. M. A. and A. De. Optimal beam splitters for the division-of-amplitude photopolarimeter. *Journal of the Optical Society of America A*, 20(5):955, 2003.

[AS05] Azzam, Rasheed M. A. and Faisal F. Sudradjat. Single-layer-coated beam splitters for the division-of-amplitude photopolarimeter. *Applied Optics*, 44(2):190, 2005.

[Azz82] R. M. A. Azzam. Division-of-amplitude Photopolarimeter (DOAP) for the Simultaneous Measurement of All Four Stokes Parameters of Light. *Optica Acta: International Journal of Optics*, 29(5):685–689, 1982.

[Fuj07] Hiroyuki Fujiwara. *Spectroscopic ellipsometry: Principles and applications*. John Wiley & Sons, Chichester and England and Hoboken and NJ, 2007.

[HMS80] P. S. Hauge, R. H. Muller, and C. G. Smith. Conventions and formulas for using the Mueller-Stokes calculus in ellipsometry. *Surface Science*, 96(1-3):81–107, 1980.

[Neg15] Christian Negara. Thickness measurement of thin films on curved surfaces with ellipsometry. In *Proceedings of the 2014 Joint Workshop of Fraunhofer IOSB and Institute for Anthropomatics, Vision and Fusion Laboratory*, Karlsruher Schriften zur Anthropomatik; 20, pages 49–65, Karlsruhe, 2015. KIT Scientific Publishing.

[NH14] Christian Negara and Matthias Hartrumpf. Ellipsometrie an gekrümmten Oberflächen. In *Forum Bildverarbeitung 2014*, pages 227–238, Karlsruhe, 2014. KIT Scientific Publishing.

[TM99] Harland G. Tompkins and William A. McGahan. *Spectroscopic ellipsometry and reflectometry: A user's guide*. Wiley, New York, 1999.

[YSZL14] Wenjia Yuan, Weidong Shen, Yueguang Zhang, and Xu Liu. Dielectric multilayer beam splitter with differential phase shift on transmission and reflection for division-of-amplitude photopolarimeter. *Optics Express*, 22(9):11011, 2014.

A Prototype System for Capturing Ground Truth Super-Resolution Data

Chengchao Qu

Vision and Fusion Laboratory
Institute for Anthropomatics and Robotics
Karlsruhe Institute of Technology (KIT), Germany
qu@kit.edu

Technical Report IES-2015-07

Abstract: Super-resolution (SR) offers an effective approach to boost quality and details of low-resolution (LR) images to obtain high-resolution (HR) images. Despite the theoretical and technical advances in the past decades, it still lacks plausible methodology to evaluate and compare different SR algorithms. The main cause to this problem lies in the missing ground truth data for SR. Unlike in many other computer vision tasks, where existing image datasets can be utilized directly, or with a little extra annotation work, SR requires that the dataset contain both LR and the corresponding HR ground truth images of the same scene captured at the same time. This work presents a novel prototype camera system to address the aforementioned difficulties of acquiring ground truth SR data. Two identical camera sensors equipped with a wide-angle lens and a telephoto lens respectively, share the same optical axis by placing a beam splitter in the optical path. The back-end program can then trigger their shutters simultaneously and precisely register the region of interests (ROIs) of the LR and HR image pairs in an automated manner free of sub-pixel interpolation. Preliminary experiments conducted on the captured face data demonstrate the special characteristics of the ground truth images compared to the simulated ones.

1 Introduction

In general, existing computer vision algorithms can only be applied to image data of standard size and quality. When the resolution of the test images goes under a certain limit, the performance is expected to drop dramatically, since resizing these low-resolution (LR) images back to a larger size alone cannot bring back the crucial high-frequency details, which are not present in the original LR images.

Straightforward solutions to the problem include adapting the employed specific algorithms to LR data [DBK06, HYBK08, PRF10], or upgrading the camera system to high-resolution (HR) models. As an alternative, though, super-resolution (SR) provides the possibility of reusing the existing data and tools. As opposed to interpolation-based methods, SR is able to recover the missing information in the original LR image by combining multiple images of the same scene, which have sub-pixel shifts among them [FREM04], or through inference of local HR structure from similar HR–LR pairs from external training data [BK02] or from the internal pyramid of the LR image itself [GBI09]. The reader is referred to [NM14, WTG+14] for an overview of state-of-the-art SR approaches.

Considering the surge of interest in SR research, datasets for evaluation purposes have received significantly less attention. Despite the fact that a huge number of datasets have been built in the computer vision society and many of them can be leveraged in various tasks [GMC+10, RDS+15], unfortunately, SR cannot take the advantage, because evaluation of SR requires a pair of HR–LR images of the same scene, one as input for the algorithms, and the other as ground truth for quantitative assessment of the output. Therefore, to the best of our knowledge, all of the previous work has made a compromise by synthetically generating the LR images using the available HR images in existing datasets, pretty much like the recently published benchmark paper [YMY14]. Nonetheless, if and how much the simulated LR image can model the complicated optical properties of the real image is yet to be justified.

On the other hand, strict conditions must be met when a new SR dataset is collected, of which the biggest challenges include temporal and spatial consistency. Thus the possibility of taking two images consecutively or the adoption of a parallel multi-camera system similar to stereo vision is eliminated, as different capturing time is not suitable for most scenes which are not completely static, and parallax of the latter setup is also not preferred for quantitative evaluation.

To circumvent these challenging requirements, a prototype of a novel dual-camera setup is proposed in this paper. The key idea is to avail of a half-silvered, semipermeable mirror, or a beam splitter, which converts the original optical path into two identical ones and redirects them towards the sensors of two identical cameras respectively. In this way, as long as the images are taken simultaneously, both the temporal and spatial prerequisites are fulfilled. The exploitation of a beam splitter is found in many optical interferometer systems, of which the most famous application is perhaps the sensor in CD/DVD/BluRay players [BLF16]. Capturing of LR and HR images is realized by a wide-angle lens and a telephoto lens mounted on the cameras respectively. Automatic image registration based on the Lukas-Kanade algorithm [LK81, BM04] returns the same region of interests (ROIs) for the pairs of images, which are experimentally analyzed in diverse aspects.

The remainder of this paper is organized as follows. The hardware setup of the proposed prototype is demonstrated in §2. After acquiring the raw image pairs with our camera system, the algorithmic details for registration and analysis of the images are discussed in §3 and §4 respectively. Following this, qualitative results on the sample data are shown in §5. Finally, we conclude our work with directions for future research in §6.

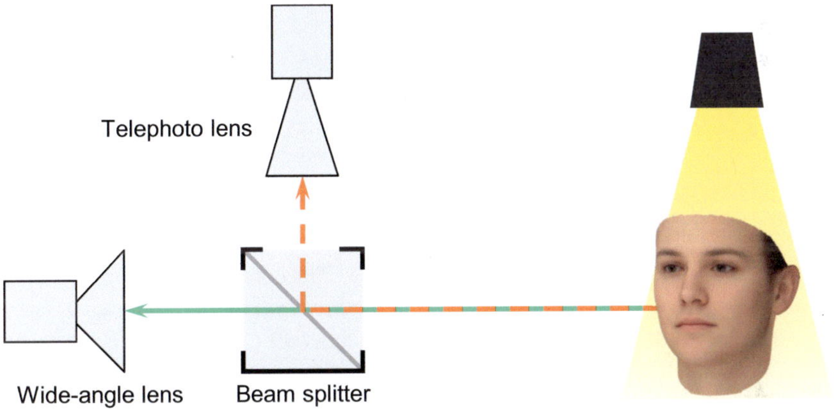

Figure 2.1: Scheme of the proposed system for capturing ground truth SR data

2 Hardware Setup

Capturing ground truth image data for evaluating SR algorithms is not a trivial task. The LR image is given as input to compute the SR result with higher resolution, which is compared with the original HR image for quantitative or qualitative assessment. Since the SR image is directly computed from the LR input, in order to conduct valid evaluation, the HR image is required to be captured exactly for the same scene at the same instant of time as that of the LR image. Some existing schemes, *e.g.*, taking the HR–LR image pairs in sequence, or on the basis of a stereo camera setup, can only partly meet the prerequisites. Violation of temporal consistency due to unsynchronized recording in the first case, and spatial consistency due to parallax in the second case, forces the method to be applicable to completely static scenes or those with a very large distance, respectively. In comparison, the novel dual-camera setup we present bypasses these limitations.

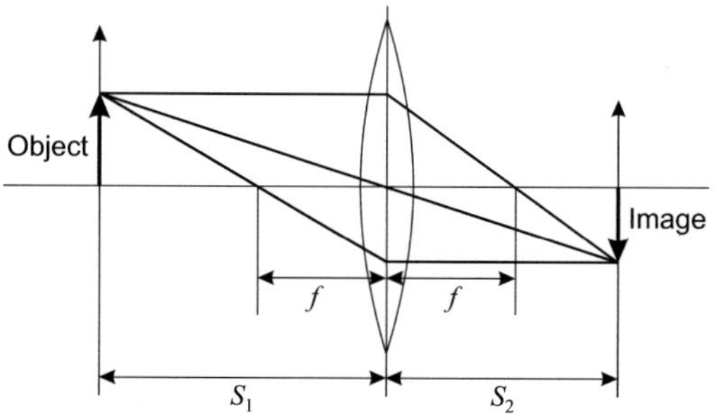

Figure 2.2: Image formation with a thin lens

The scheme of the system is depicted in Fig. 2.1. The core idea is the introduction of a semipermeable mirror into the optical path, which splits the incident light from the scene in two. This can be realized with a half-silvered mirror, or in our case, a beam splitter with 50:50 split ratio. Its common form is a cube with two halves of triangular glass prisms glued together using resin or the like. When the light beam enters through the entrance face of the cube to the glue layer, half of the light is reflected and the rest is transmitted through the prisms on account of total internal reflection within the layer. In our prototype system, a beam splitter with 50:50 split ratio is deployed. Two identical cameras are directed at the exit faces of the beam splitter and the cameras are equipped with a wide-angle lens and a telephoto lens respectively, such that the one camera with larger field of view (FOV) captures a larger scene with lower resolution, and the other camera with smaller FOV captures zoomed HR details.

The upcoming problem is the choice of lenses and the positions of the cameras to achieve the desired magnification factor for the HR–LR image pairs in SR. According to the thin lens formula [Hec01] depicted in Fig. 2.2, magnification factor m_{Object}, *i.e.*, the size of the image in proportion to the size of the original object is

$$m_{\text{Object}} = -\frac{S_2}{S_1} = \frac{f}{f - S_1} = \frac{f - S_2}{f},$$

where f denotes the focal length of the lens, and S_1 and S_2 are the distances from the lens center to the object and the image respectively. For the magnification factor m_{SR} which we are more interested in, the following approximation applies

$$m_{\mathrm{SR}} = \frac{f_{\mathrm{HR}}}{f_{\mathrm{HR}} - S_1} \Big/ \frac{f_{\mathrm{LR}}}{f_{\mathrm{LR}} - S_1} \approx \frac{f_{\mathrm{HR}}}{f_{\mathrm{LR}}}, \tag{2.1}$$

where the object distance is similar for both cameras and much larger than the focal length, *i.e.*, $S_1 \gg f$. On the other side, since m_{Object} for non-macro lenses is very small, one has $S_2 \approx f$, then from Fig. 2.2, the camera positions can be determined by

$$S_{2,\mathrm{HR}} - S_{2,\mathrm{LR}} = f_{\mathrm{HR}} - f_{\mathrm{LR}}, \tag{2.2}$$

when the focal lengths for HR and LR cameras are approximately computed by Eq. (2.1) for the given magnification factor m_{SR}.

However, by virtue of the complex optical elements in real objectives, the thin lens approximation does not always apply. As a consequence, Eqs. (2.1) and (2.2) do not necessarily hold. Instead of employing prime lenses with the exact fixed focal lengths from Eq. (2.1), zoom lenses are utilized as a workaround, so that the true focal lengths and camera positions can be fine-tuned in the proximity of the theoretical values. An interactive adjustment process is presented in §3.

The built prototype system for the scheme in Fig. 2.1 is illustrated in Fig. 2.3. A 50:50 beam splitter for visible light in the range of 400–700 nm is located at the intersection of the two camera axes. The C-mount cameras possess a relatively large 1/1.2″ CMOS sensor with merely 2 megapixels (1920×1200), which allows for higher signal-to-noise ratio (SNR) thanks to larger pixel size. An ultra-wide angle 4.8 mm f/1.8 prime lens, which serves as the LR lens, and a 12.5–75 mm f/1.2 zoom lens for the HR images are mounted on each camera. The 6× zoom ratio is ideal to experiment with different magnification factors m_{SR}. The large aperture of both lenses is also fast enough for low-light indoor scenarios. In order to mitigate in-plane rotational discrepancy between the pair of images, one camera is installed on a kinetic mounting surface for pitch and roll adjustment.

In summary, the final prototype is able to account for scaling and rotation in the registration process, leaving only the translational offset to be determined algorithmically. As such, concerns that a posterior compensation in scaling and rotation with interpolation could deteriorate the original image quality are addressed.

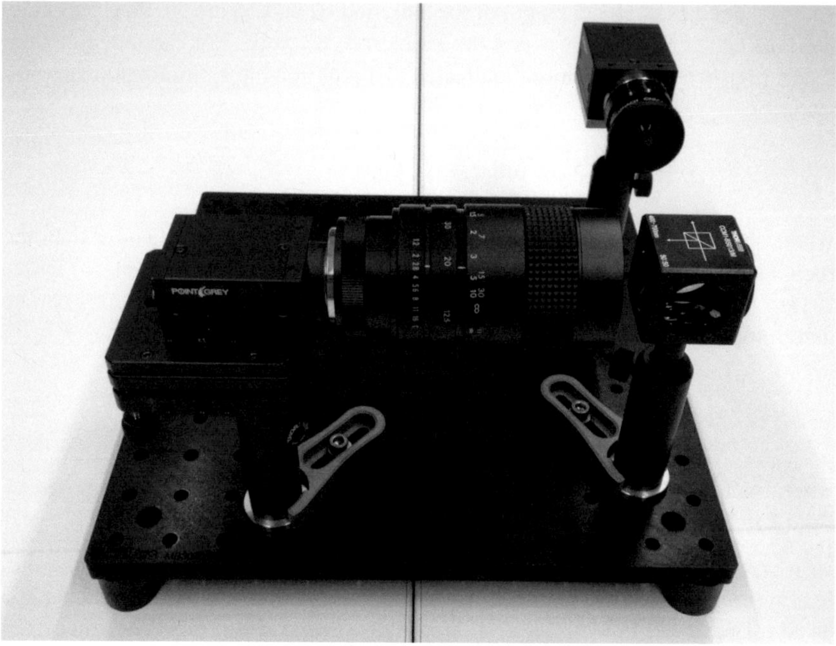

Figure 2.3: Prototype of the proposed system for capturing ground truth SR data

3 Image Registration

The hardware prototype in §2 performs a rough presetting of the desired SR ground truth capturing workflow. Raw HR–LR image pairs with approximately the desired magnification factor can be acquired. However, further processing must be done, before the images are ready for the evaluation purpose. Since the HR image covers only a small region in the center of the corresponding LR image, the surrounding irrelevant part should be filtered out. In the meantime, fine-tuning of the magnification factor m_{SR} obtained in Eq. (2.1) can also be conducted during the registration procedure.

Given a coarse alignment in scaling and rotation from the hardware system, only translational motion needs to be estimated, which greatly reduces the degree of freedom (DOF) and computational complexity to exploit the classical but yet powerful Lukas-Kanade algorithm [Sze11, LK81, BM04]. The objective is to obtain the update $\mathbf{\Delta}\boldsymbol{\theta}$ of the parametrized motion $\boldsymbol{\theta}$ by minimizing the sum of squared differences (SSD) between the fixed template $\mathbf{T}$ and moving image $\mathbf{I}$

$$\sum_{\boldsymbol{\xi}} \|\mathbf{I}(\mathbf{W}(\boldsymbol{\xi};\boldsymbol{\theta}+\mathbf{\Delta}\boldsymbol{\theta})) - \mathbf{T}(\boldsymbol{\xi})\|_2^2$$

subject to warping $\mathbf{W}(\boldsymbol{\xi};\boldsymbol{\theta})$ of the pixels $\boldsymbol{\xi}$ [LK81]. Leveraging Taylor series expansion and the partial derivatives with respect to $\boldsymbol{\theta}$, closed-form solution can be obtained. Later, it is proved that performing inverse update on the template $\mathbf{T}$ instead of $\mathbf{I}$

$$\sum_{\boldsymbol{\xi}} \|\mathbf{I}(\mathbf{W}(\boldsymbol{\xi};\boldsymbol{\theta})) - \mathbf{T}(\mathbf{W}(\boldsymbol{\xi};\mathbf{\Delta}\boldsymbol{\theta}))\|_2^2$$

can substantially boost the efficiency, as the inverse Hessian and steepest descent images can be precomputed at the initial $(\boldsymbol{\xi};\mathbf{0})$ instead of the current iteration $(\boldsymbol{\xi};\boldsymbol{\theta})$ [BM04].

Concretely, with a pair of HR–LR images, we first set our template $\mathbf{T}$ as the center of the LR image, or as the ROI detected by some algorithm (*e.g.*, faces by [VJ04]). The moving image $\mathbf{I}$ to be aligned is obtained by downsampling the HR image with the desired magnification factor m_{SR}. The initial translation $\boldsymbol{\theta}_t^{(0)}$ for $\mathbf{I}$ is set as the HR image, or again based on the localized ROI. Subsequently, continuous Lukas-Kanade translational registration is conducted and the result error image is shown to the user. After manual tuning of tip and tilt on the kinetic platform and the focal length f_{HR} for the HR camera, precise alignment of HR–LR image pairs without any sub-pixel interpolation is computed. The whole image registration procedure is summarized in Alg. 3.1.

4 Image Analysis

In SR, the observation model of the conventional image acquisition process turns an HR image $\mathbf{x}$ of dimension $m_{\mathrm{SR}}N_1 \times m_{\mathrm{SR}}N_2$ into the captured LR image $\mathbf{z}$ of dimension $N_1 \times N_2$ with

$$\mathbf{z} = (\mathbf{B}_{\mathbf{k}} \circ \mathbf{W}_{\boldsymbol{\theta}}(\mathbf{x})) \downarrow_{m_{\mathrm{SR}}} + \mathbf{n}, \tag{4.1}$$

where $\mathbf{W}$ first warps the original scene via the parametrized motion $\boldsymbol{\theta}$. Then $\mathbf{B}$ models the blurring effect by the $K \times K$ kernel $\mathbf{k}$ and $\downarrow_{m_{\mathrm{SR}}}$ denotes decimation with factor m_{SR}. The additive system noise, often assumed to be white with zero-mean Gaussian distribution, is represented by $\mathbf{n}$. The objective of SR is to

Algorithm 3.1 Interactive HR–LR image registration

Input: Roughly registered HR–LR image pair
Output: Precisely registered HR–LR image pair

Initialize ROIs for HR and LR images
Crop template $\mathbf{T}$ from the LR image
Shrink the HR image with factor m_{SR} as image $\mathbf{I}$
Initialize translation $\boldsymbol{\theta}_t^{(0)}$ for $\mathbf{I}$
while not aligned **do**
  Compute $\boldsymbol{\theta}_t$ using Lukas-Kanade algorithm
  Crop $\mathbf{I}$ based on $\boldsymbol{\theta}_t$
  Compare error image of $\mathbf{T}$ and cropped $\mathbf{I}$
  if in-plane rotation not aligned **then**
    Adjust tip and tilt of the kinetic platform
  end if
  if magnification not aligned **then**
    Adjust f_{HR}
  end if
end while

reversely model the image formation process in Eq. (4.1) given the LR image $\mathbf{z}$, which is an ill-posed problem with only the subsampling factor m_{SR} being known. Hence extra knowledge from internal or external sources is required [NM14, WTG$^+$14].

In this work, since both the ground truth HR–LR image pairs $\mathbf{x}$ and $\mathbf{z}$ are captured and the motion $\boldsymbol{\theta}$ is compensated by the image registration process in §3, analysis of the images is a lot easier compared to SR, which simplifies Eq. (4.1) into

$$\mathbf{z} = (\mathbf{k} * \mathbf{x}) \downarrow_{m_{\text{SR}}} + \mathbf{n}, \tag{4.2}$$

where $*$ denotes 2D-convolution. Manipulation of Eq. (4.2) must be performed to convert both of the intractable operators into matrix multiplication to allow for further calculation

$$\text{vec}(\mathbf{z}) = \mathbf{S}_{m_{\text{SR}}} \mathbf{T}_{\mathbf{x}} \, \text{vec}(\mathbf{k}_{\text{mirror}}) + \text{vec}(\mathbf{n}),$$

where the square blurring kernel $\mathbf{k}$ is mirrored and vectorized by $\text{vec}(\mathbf{k}_{\text{mirror}}) \in \mathbb{R}^{K^2}$. $\mathbf{T}_{\mathbf{x}}$ vectorizes each $K \times K$ sliding window in the HR image $\mathbf{x}$ as a row vector and stacks them in vertical direction, yielding a $m_{\text{SR}}^2 N_1 N_2 \times K^2$ matrix. As such, the 2D-convolution is replaced exactly by a matrix multiplication. Finally, $\mathbf{S}_{m_{\text{SR}}} \in \mathbb{Z}^{N_1 N_2 \times m_{\text{SR}}^2 N_1 N_2}$ is a sparse mapping matrix to shrink the HR image to LR using nearest neighbor, *i.e.*, for each LR pixel represented by the row i in $\mathbf{S}_{m_\mathrm{SR}}$, only column j corresponding to the selected HR pixel is set to one.

Assuming independent noise $\mathbf{n}$ with uniform variance facilitates straightforward least squares solution of the blurring kernel $\mathbf{k}$ with maximum-likelihood estimation (MLE) by minimizing the SSD

$$\|\mathbf{S}_{m_\mathrm{SR}} \mathbf{T}_\mathbf{x} \operatorname{vec}(\mathbf{k}_\mathrm{mirror}) - \operatorname{vec}(\mathbf{z})\|_2^2,$$

which can also be found in blind deconvolution [LWDF11]. A globally optimal solution for the kernel exists by solving for the convex quadratic programming problem [NW06] in the form of

$$\min_\mathbf{y} \|\mathbf{A}\mathbf{y} - \mathbf{b}\|_2^2 = \min_\mathbf{y} \mathbf{y}^\top \mathbf{A}^\top \mathbf{A}\mathbf{y} - 2\mathbf{b}^\top \mathbf{A}\mathbf{y} + c.$$

Imposing non-negative and unit ℓ_1-norm constraints ensures a valid estimate of the blurring kernel. Optionally to resemble Gaussian kernels, additional symmetry constraint is applicable.

5 Experiments

The presented camera system is deployed in an indoor environment to take sample HR–LR images for evaluation. The most commonly used magnification factor $m_\mathrm{SR} = 4$ is chosen as in the survey [NM14]. Accordingly, the focal length for the HR lens f_HR and the relative camera positions are initialized based on Eqs. (2.1) and (2.2) respectively. Subsequently, Alg. 3.1 takes care of interactive hardware tuning and cropping of the registered HR–LR pairs. A face detector [VJ04] is employed to automatically extract the ROIs from the captured raw image pairs.

An example of the captured and registered images is illustrated in Fig. 5.1. By dropping the outer region of the LR image, the FOV in Fig. 5.1(b) is roughly equivalent to the HR image in Fig. 5.1(a) with 1/4 of the pixels in both dimensions. The resulting LR face has a width of approximately 30 pixels, covering only the central 1.5% of the total 1920 pixels, which is critical to diminish distortion and chromatic aberration of the 4.8 mm ultra-wide angle lens.

We recover the blurring kernels with the techniques introduced in §4 and the results are demonstrated in Fig. 5.2. Because the kernels in Fig. 5.2(b) do not impose any further constraints, they are considered to be optimal for the given

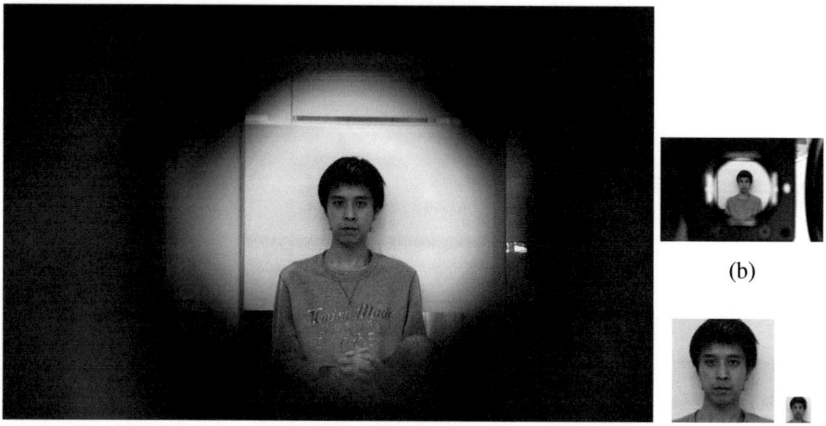

(a) (b) (c) (d)

Figure 5.1: An example pair of (a) HR and (b) LR images captured by the prototype system with cropped (c) HR and (d) LR ROIs

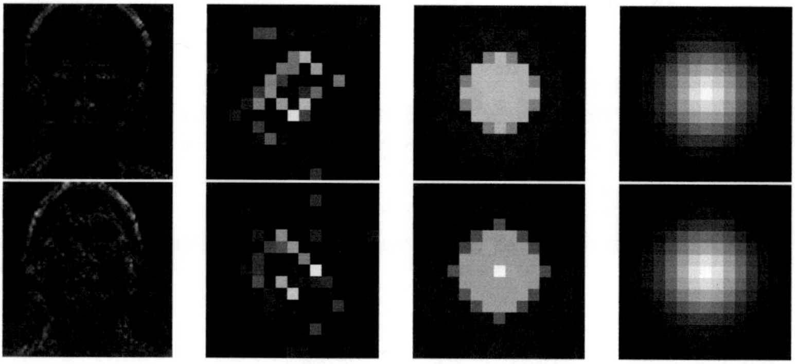

(a) (b) (c) (d)

Figure 5.2: Results analyzed on two sample HR–LR image pairs: (a) the error images between the LR images and the HR images blurred with the recovered kernels without symmetry constraint in (b) and downsampled, (c) the recovered kernels with symmetry constraint, (d) the Gaussian kernel with the lowest HR–LR reconstruction errors

HR–LR image pair. At first sight, it is obvious that the registration process integrating hardware and algorithmic solutions reveals nearly perfect precision in both magnification and translational offset. Solely at the boundary of the hair, where aliasing effect could happen in LR images, more visible error can be seen (see Fig. 5.2(a)). Furthermore, the true blurring kernels are far from the widely applied Gaussian kernels. Even by enforcing symmetry constraint in quadratic programming, the recovered kernels in Fig. 5.2(c) do not resemble the Gaussian in Fig. 5.2(d) with the best kernel width $\sigma = 2.4$ in terms of reconstruction error. The importance of true ground truth SR data and reliable blurring kernel estimation for SR algorithms hereby justify the contribution of this work.

6 Conclusions and Future Work

The problem of acquiring ground truth SR datasets is addressed in this paper. A dual-camera imaging system featuring a beam splitter to allow for capturing of HR and LR images with temporal and spatial synchronization is proposed. An interactive process is presented for the nontrivial pixel-accurate registration of the HR–LR image pairs. The necessity of such ground truth data for SR is confirmed by the analysis of the image characteristics.

The SR community has paid relatively less attention to the effect of blurring kernel. Those that do often assume Gaussian kernels with the width known a priori. It is proved in [EGA$^+$13] that this problem actually matters. Our future work will focus on building a larger SR dataset with the prototype system and conducting systematical evaluation of kernel and noise properties to spur more interest for these important aspects.

Bibliography

[BK02] S. Baker and T. Kanade. Limits on super-resolution and how to break them. *IEEE Trans. Pattern Anal. Mach. Intell.*, 24(9):1167–1183, 2002.

[BLF16] J. Beyerer, F. P. León, and C. Frese. Methods of image acquisition. In *Machine Vision*, pages 223–365. Springer Berlin Heidelberg, 2016.

[BM04] S. Baker and I. Matthews. Lucas-Kanade 20 years on: A unifying framework. *Int. J. Comput. Vis.*, 56(3):221–255, 2004.

[DBK06] G. Dedeoğlu, S. Baker, and T. Kanade. Resolution-aware fitting of active appearance models to low-resolution images. In *ECCV*, volume 2, pages 83–97, 2006.

[EGA$^+$13] N. Efrat, D. Glasner, A. Apartsin, B. Nadler, and A. Levin. Accurate blur models vs. image priors in single image super-resolution. In *ICCV*, pages 2832–2839, 2013.

[FREM04] S. Farsiu, M. D. Robinson, M. Elad, and P. Milanfar. Fast and robust multiframe super resolution. *IEEE Trans. Image Process.*, 13(10):1327–1344, 2004.

[GBI09] D. Glasner, S. Bagon, and M. Irani. Super-resolution from a single image. In *CVPR*, pages 349–356, 2009.

[GMC+10] R. Gross, I. Matthews, J. Cohn, T. Kanade, and S. Baker. Multi-PIE. *Image Vis. Comput.*, 28(5):807–813, 2010.

[Hec01] E. Hecht. *Optics*. Addison Wesley, 4 edition, 2001.

[HYBK08] P. H. Hennings-Yeomans, S. Baker, and B. V. K. V. Kumar. Simultaneous super-resolution and feature extraction for recognition of low-resolution faces. In *CVPR*, pages 1–8, 2008.

[LK81] B. D. Lucas and T. Kanade. An iterative image registration technique with an application to stereo vision. In *IJCAI*, volume 2, pages 674–679, 1981.

[LWDF11] A. Levin, Y. Weiss, F. Durand, and W. T. Freeman. Efficient marginal likelihood optimization in blind deconvolution. In *CVPR*, pages 2657–2664, 2011.

[NM14] K. Nasrollahi and T. B. Moeslund. Super-resolution: a comprehensive survey. *Mach. Vis. Appl.*, 25(6):1423–1468, 2014.

[NW06] J. Nocedal and S. J. Wright. *Numerical Optimization*. Springer New York, 2 edition, 2006.

[PRF10] D. Park, D. Ramanan, and C. Fowlkes. Multiresolution models for object detection. In *ECCV*, pages 241–254, 2010.

[RDS+15] O. Russakovsky, J. Deng, H. Su, J. Krause, S. Satheesh, S. Ma, Z. Huang, A. Karpathy, A. Khosla, M. Bernstein, A. C. Berg, and F.-F. Li. ImageNet large scale visual recognition challenge. *Int. J. Comput. Vis.*, 115(3):211–252, 2015.

[Sze11] R. Szeliski. Dense motion estimation. In *Computer Vision: Algorithms and Applications*, pages 335–374. Springer London, 2011.

[VJ04] P. Viola and M. J. Jones. Robust real-time face detection. *Int. J. Comput. Vis.*, 57(2):137–154, 2004.

[WTG+14] N. Wang, D. Tao, X. Gao, X. Li, and J. Li. A comprehensive survey to face hallucination. *Int. J. Comput. Vis.*, 106(1):9–30, 2014.

[YMY14] C.-Y. Yang, C. Ma, and M.-H. Yang. Single-image super-resolution: A benchmark. In *ECCV*, pages 372–386, 2014.

Overview on Machine Vision Methods for Finding Defects in Transparent Objects

Johannes Meyer

Vision and Fusion Laboratory
Institute for Anthropomatics
Karlsruhe Institute of Technology (KIT), Germany
johannes.meyer@kit.edu

Technical Report IES-2015-08

Abstract: Machine vision methods are widely and successfully used for assuring the quality of any produced goods. Many of these methods require the test object's surface to be either nearly Lambertian or specular. Since transparent materials do not meet these requirements, suitable approaches for the inspection of transparent materials are needed. This paper provides an overview on existing methods for testing transparent objects for enclosed impurities, defects affecting the shape or anomalies of the index of refraction. Besides, possible topics for conducting further research are identified.

1 Introduction

Transparent materials play an important role in many fields of industries. They are often used in tasks or to create products that require high material quality and reliability, e.g., windshields for aircrafts and automobiles or high-precision optical elements like lenses used for guiding laser beams in medical surgery applications [Mey14]. Therefore, it is a common visual inspection task to check transparent objects for (enclosed) contaminants like absorbing particles (e.g., dust), scattering structures (e.g., air bubbles, surface scratches) or defects affecting the macroscopic 3D-geometry. For many applications, also the homogeneity of the material's refractive index is of utter importance. However, it cannot be evaluated by the naked human eye since it is not capable of observing phase effects. In general, the visual inspection of transparent objects is a fatiguing task for humans.

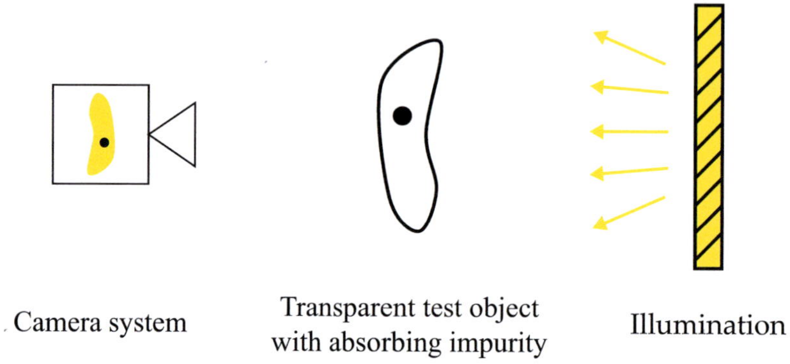

Figure 2.1: Conventional transmission inspection setup: An undirected light source illuminates the test object from one side. The transmitted light is observed by a camera system from the other side. Absorbing defects present in the test object appear as dark structures in the camera image.

The risk that the inspector oversees a material flaw increases notably after a small period of inspection time. This clarifies the importance of automated methods for the visual inspection of transparent objects.

There are many elaborated methods for inspecting opaque or specular objects. However, these methods are not applicable to transparent objects, for example, the laser lines employed by many active pattern projection systems cannot be observed on the test objects surface due to its transparency. Research has been performed to develop inspection methods suitable for transparent objects. This paper reviews the research results of the past years with respect to the automated testing of transparent objects for absorbing or scattering impurities, surface flaws, defects affecting the object's macroscopic 3D-geometry and for anomalies of the index of refraction. Since many of the reviewed methods follow an individual and complex approach they are described in dedicated sections.

2 Transmission setup

In common transmission setups for visual inspection, an undirected light source illuminates the test object from one side and a camera system observes the transmitted radiation on the test object's other side (see Fig. 2.1) [BLF15, ANW$^+$09].

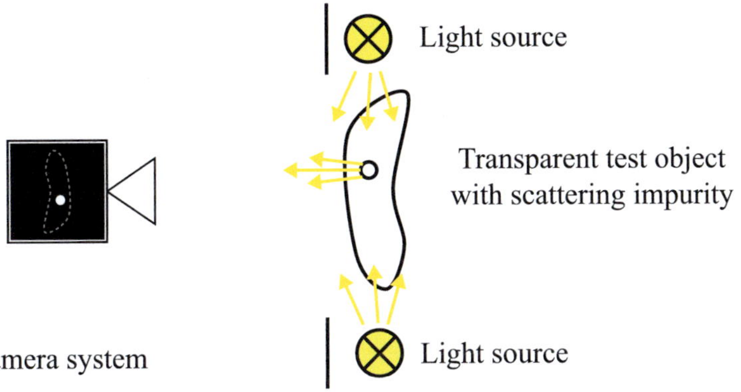

Figure 3.1: Conventional dark field inspection setup: One or more light sources, which are not in the camera's view, illuminate the test object. Any scattering impurity inside or on the test object will scatter some light into the camera and will result in bright structures in the observed image.

If the camera is focused on the test object, such setups are able to visualize absorbing contaminants. However, depending on the object's shape and index of refraction, some parts of the test object might not be inspected because the illuminating light rays can partly miss the camera [Hec13]. The setup cannot visualize scattering defects as – due to the undirected illumination – the light rays that miss the camera because of the scattering will not lead to a local intensity drop since other rays with another angle of incidence are likely to be scattered into the camera instead.

3 Dark field setup

In dark field setups the test object is usually illuminated in such a way, that in the case of a defect-free test object, no light reaches the camera (see Fig. 3.1). So, a defect-free test object results in a dark inspection image. Conversely, any scattering defect present in the transparent object will scatter the incident light into multiple directions – especially into the camera [BLF15, ANW$^+$09, Hec13].

In general, dark field illumination is also capable of visualizing surface flaws like scratches. However, defects affecting the macroscopic 3D-geometry or inhomogeneities of the object's index of refraction cannot be visualized.

4 Retroreflection system

In order to overcome the limitations of the transmission setup (see Sect. 2) regarding test objects of complex geometry and with a high index of refraction, Hartrumpf et al. proposed an approach – the so-called Purity system [HH09, HVLS08, MLP$^+$10] – that employs a retroreflective foil. Besides, their approach is able to simultaneously capture a dark field illuminated image by means of color multiplexing the different illumination sources.

Figure 4.1 shows a sketch of the respective optical setup. For obtaining the transmission image, a bright field illumination shines onto the test object out of the camera's direction via a beam splitter. The retroreflector – which is placed behind the test object – reflects any incident light ray back into its original direction. Since the Helmholtz reciprocity principle [Hec13] holds, the retroreflector compensates the refraction effect occuring at the interface between the transparentn object and the surrounding medium. This is why the Purity system is also capable of inspecting test objects having a complex geometry or a high index of refraction.

Besides the common dark field illumination described in Sect. 3, the approach uses an additional dark field illumination that shines on the test object with an angle of incidence that is close to Brewster's angle. This illumination visualizes small scattering contaminants located on the test object's surface. By employing individual colors (red, green, blue) for the different illumination components, a single acquired color camera image contains the information of all three illumination setups in separate channels.

Although it can capture absorbing or scattering impurities and surface flaws, the Purity system is not capable of visualizing defects affecting the test object's macroscopic 3D-geometry or its index of refraction. However, since the resulting inspection images require only simple image processing routines, the method's implementation is suitable for real-time applications.

5 Structured illumination system

In order to check complex-shaped transparent objects, e.g., headlamp lenses of automobiles, for absorbing or scattering impurities and for surface defects, Martínez et al. employ a robotic platform that moves a so-called 'binary active lighting system' around the test object [MOGG12]. Their illumination approach uses a monitor displaying a moving binary black and white stripe pattern (see

Fig. 5.1). They require the test object to have no cavities and that the front and back surface are parallel to each other. Any scattering defect on or inside the test object will result in a deflection of rays. The deflection causes that some light of a displayed bright strips produces a bright spot in the camera image of one of the adjacent dark stripes (see Fig. 5.2). Conversely, an absorbing defect will result in a dark structure in the image of the corresponding bright stripe. By phase shifting the binary pattern and capturing multiple images, the test object is successively scanned.

Because of the robot platform, the setup can inspect even objects with a complex 3D-geometry. However, a sensor planning strategy has to be found for every type of test object. The proposed approach is not capable of visualizing defects affecting the macroscopic 3D-geometry of the object or its index of refraction.

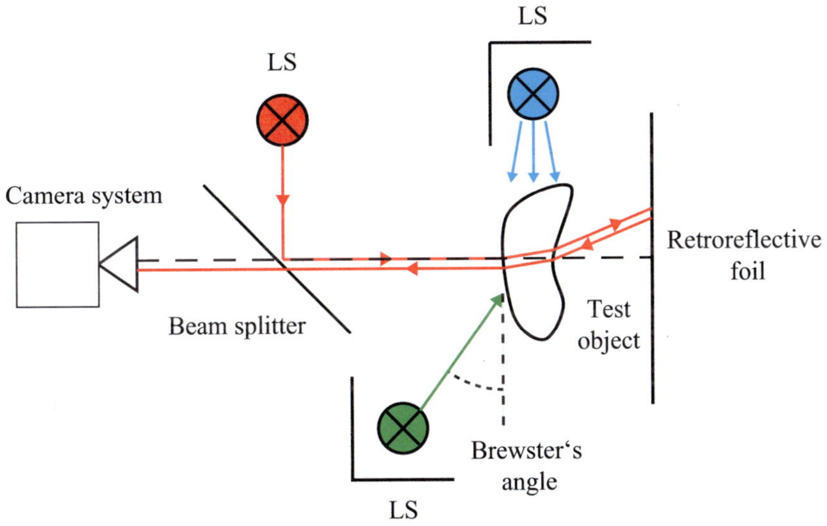

Figure 4.1: Setup of the Purity system: Via a beam splitter, the test object is illuminated from the direction of the camera's optical axis (red). A retroreflective foil placed behind the test object mitigates refraction effects occurring at the interfaces between the test object and the surrounding medium. A dark field illumination (blue) visualizes scattering defects. A third light source (green) illuminates the test object under Brewster's angle in order to visualize surface contaminants, e.g., dust particles.

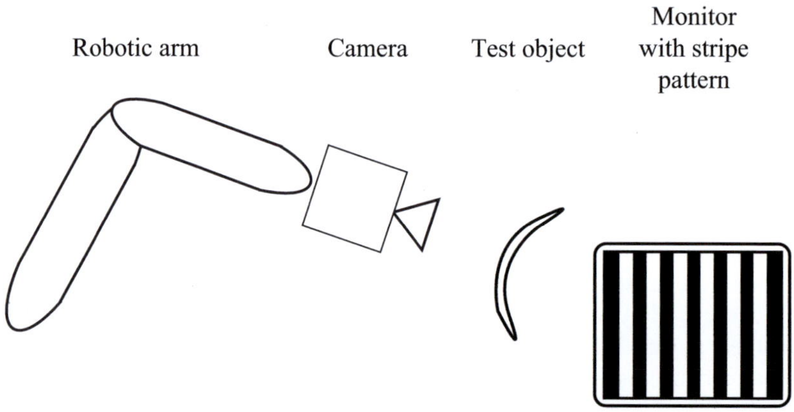

Figure 5.1: Structured illumination setup: A monitor realizes the 'binary active lighting system' and illuminates the test object. A camera observes the transmitted light. In order to inspect the whole test object, a robotic arm moves the camera to precomputed positions.

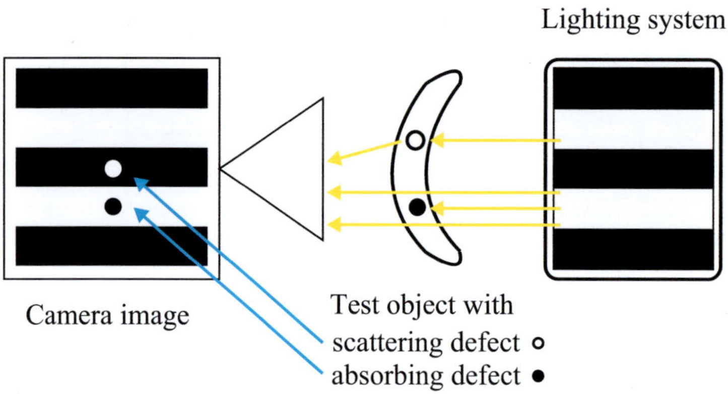

Figure 5.2: Defect visualization by means of the 'binary active lighting system': Absorbing defects are imaged to dark structures if illuminated by a bright stripe. Scattering defects are visualized by causing bright regions in the images of adjacent black stripes.

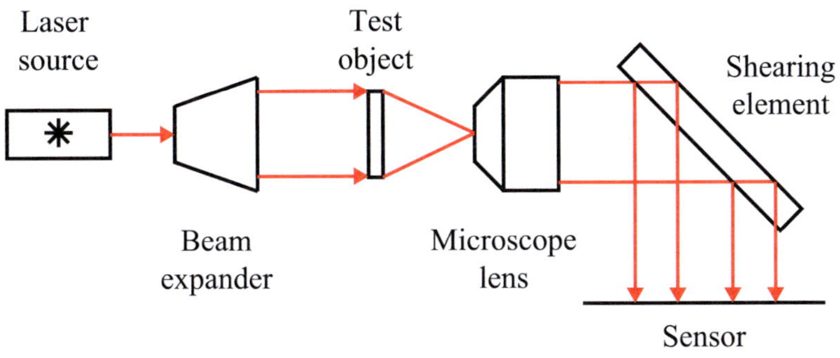

Figure 6.1: Transmissive optical shearing interferometer: An expanded coherent laser beam illuminates the test object. The transmitted light is collected by a microscope lens that magnifies the test object. A shearing element tilted by 90° directs the light onto a sensor, where the reflections from the shearing element's front and back surface interfere with each other. The resulting hologram is captured by the sensor.

6 Transmissive optical shearing interferometer

Seo et al. employ digital holographic microscopy in order to detect surface scratches on transparent cover glasses with a magnitude of less than 10^{-6} m [SKKK14, SKK14]. Their proposed setup is based on a transmission-type optical shearing interferometer as shown in Fig. 6.1.

An expanded coherent laser beam illuminates the test object. The transmitted light is collected by a microscope lens and directed onto a shearing element, i.e., a high-quality glass-plate with a thickness smaller than the laser's coherence length. The reflections from the front and back surface create hologram patterns on the sensor by interfering with each other.

By acquiring two holograms – one with the inserted test object and one without it – the thickness of the investigated object can be reconstructed and can reveal surface scratches.

Although the author has only applied the presented approach to find defects affecting the test object's surface structure, it should also be appropriate to detect inhomogeneities of the index of refraction. However, the method cannot visualize absorbing or scattering impurities and defects affecting the macroscopic 3D-geometry.

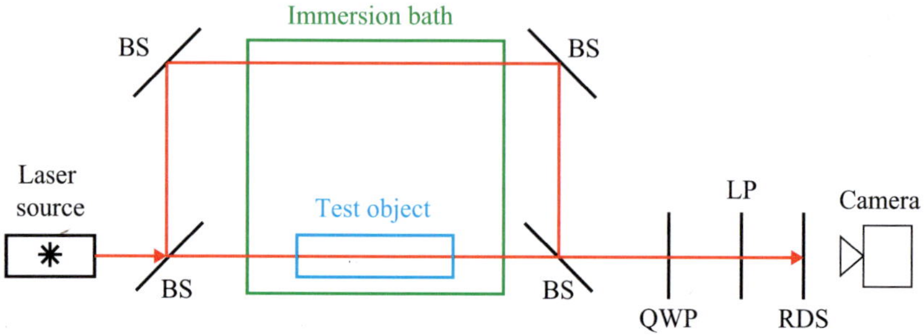

Figure 7.1: Phase shifting interferometer: A coherent laser beam is split into a reference arm (upper path) and a probe arm (lower path) by a polarizing beam splitter (BS). The probe arm passes the test object that is immersed in a liquid matching the test object's index of refraction. Another beam splitter recombines the two arms. A quarter-wave plate (QWP) and a rotatable linear polarizer induce an adjustable phase shift to the transmitted beam. A camera observes the interference pattern created by the two beams on a rotating diffuser screen.

7 Phase shifting interferometer

Chatterjee used a polarization phase shifting interferometer in order to test high-quality optical glass slabs for inhomogeneities of the local distribution of the index of refraction [Cha15]. An expanded laser beam is split into a reference arm and a probe arm. The test object is immersed into a liquid that matches the object's index of refraction. After the probe beam traversed the test object, it passes a quarter-wave plate and a rotatable linear polarizer together with the reference beam. In concert, the two beams create an interference pattern on a rotating diffuser screen that is used to reduce speckle. The screen is observed by a camera. Figure 7.1 shows the principle optical inspection setup.

By employing polarizing beam splitters and the quarter-wave plate, an adjustable phase-shift can be induced by rotating the linear polarizer. Capturing and processing images for different rotation angles of the linear polarizer allows to unwrap the phase information of the optical path difference conveyed in the interference patterns. The unwrapped phase can be used to detect inhomogeneities of the index of refraction with an accuracy of 10^{-6}.

	Absorbing impurities	Scattering impurities	Shape flaws	Macr.3D-geometry	Index of refraction
Transmission	+	-	-	-	-
Dark field	-	+	+	-	-
Retroreflection	+	+	+	-	-
Structured illumination	+	+	+	-	-
Shearing interferometer	-	-	+	-	-
Phase shifting interferometer	-	-	-	-	+

Table 8.1: Summary of the different approaches for defect visualization in transparent objects. +: the type of defect is visualized; -: the type of defect is not visualized.

8 Conclusion and future work

This contribution discussed some of the recent works regarding the automated visual inspection of transparent objects. Table 8.1 lists the covered methods and summarizes their suitability for industrial inspection applications.

Each of the presented approaches is capable of visualizing one or more of the considered defect types but none of them is sensitive to them all. Therefore, a possible topic for future research could be to find an inspection method that is able to capture all mentioned defect types.

Besides, industrial inspection tasks often pose challenging timing conditions that cannot be met by some of the discussed approaches. Hence, improving the image acquisition and processing speed of automated inspection methods for transparent objects represents another open research question.

Bibliography

[ANW+09] Gil Abramovich, Christopher Nafis, Yana Williams, Kevin Harding, and Eric Tkaczyk. Three-dimensional embedded defect detection and localization in a semi-transparent medium. In *Proc. SPIE*, volume 7432, page 74321C, 2009.

[BLF15] Jürgen. Beyerer, Fernando Puente León, and Christian Frese. *Machine Vision: Automated Visual Inspection: Theory, Practice and Applications.* Springer Berlin Heidelberg, 2015.

[Cha15] Sanjib Chatterjee. Determination of refractive index in-homogeneity of transparent, isotropic optical materials. In *Advances in Optical Science and Engineering*, pages 61–66. Springer, 2015.

[Hec13] Eugene Hecht. *Optics*. Pearson, San Francisco, 4th edition, 2013.

[HH09] Matthias Hartrumpf and Rüdiger Heintz. Device and method for the classification of transparent components in a material flow. Patent WO 2009/049594 A1, 2009.

[HVLS08] Matthias Hartrumpf, Kai-Uwe Vieth, Thomas Längle, and Günter Struck. Neues Verfahren zur Sichtprüfung transparenter Materialien. In *Sensorgestützte Sortierung*, pages 57–58, Aachen, March 2008. Gesellschaft für Bergbau, Metallurgie, Rohstoff- und Umwelttechnik.

[Mey14] Johannes Meyer. Visual inspection of transparent objects – physical basics, existing methods and novel ideas. Technical Report IES-2014-04, Karlsruhe Institute of Technology, 2014.

[MLP+10] Wolfgang Melchert, Thomas Längle, Philipp Pätzold, Robin Gruna, and Michael Palmer. Automatische Sichtprüfung strukturierter transparenter Materialien. In *Forum Bildverarbeitung, F. Puente León und M. Heizmann, Hrsg., Regensburg, Germany*, pages 143–153, 2010.

[MOGG12] S Satorres Martínez, J Gómez Ortega, J Gámez García, and A Sánchez García. A machine vision system for defect characterization on transparent parts with non-plane surfaces. *Machine Vision and Applications*, 23(1):1–13, 2012.

[SKK14] Kwang-Beom Seo, Byung-Mok Kim, and Eun-Soo Kim. Digital holographic microscopy based on a modified lateral shearing interferometer for three-dimensional visual inspection of nanoscale defects on transparent objects. *Nanoscale research letters*, 9(1):1–14, 2014.

[SKKK14] Kwang-Beom Seo, Byung-Mok Kim, Jung-Sik Koo, and Eun-Soo Kim. A novel three-dimensional visual inspection scheme for defect detection of transparent materials based on the digital holographic microscopy. In *International Multidisciplinary Microscopy Congress*, pages 37–44. Springer, 2014.

Towards Graphical Partially Observable Monte-Carlo Planning

Julius Pfrommer

Vision and Fusion Laboratory
Institute for Anthropomatics
Karlsruhe Institute of Technology (KIT), Germany
julius.pfrommer@kit.edu

Technical Report IES-2015-09

Abstract: Sample-based online algorithms are state of the art for solving Partially Observable Markov Decision Problems (POMDP). But also the state of the art solver POMCP still suffers from the curse of dimensionality and curse of history. In Distributed POMDP, independent agents jointly optimise their actions under some coordination mechanism where every agent has access to a subset of the observations. In this work, we introduce Graphical POMDP (GPOMDP) drawing from existing Distributed POMDP appraoches as well as graph-based formulations as found in graphical probabilistic models. Further, we propose the Graphical POMCP (GPOMCP) algorithm that combines POMCP with message passing similar to the Belief Propagation (BP) algorithm from Graphical Probabilistic Models. In preliminary tests, GPOMCP shows good performance on a common Distributed POMDP benchmark.

1 Introduction

Partially Observable Markov Decision Problems (POMDP) [KLC98] capture planning scenarios with both nondeterministic system dynamics and uncertainty about the current state. The Partially Observable Monte-Carlo Planning (POMCP) algorithm [SV10] is a current state of the art technique for solving POMDP. On some benchmarks, it led to several magnitudes of speed improvements compared to previous point-based planning methods such as SARSOP [KHL08]. A recent publication by Amato and Oliehoek [AO15] applies POMCP to Distributed POMDP in the Dec-POMDP model. In this technical report, we present preliminary findings on a novel variation of POMCP for Distributed

POMDP where value estimates are propagated in a graph structure representing a decomposition of the POMDP. The resulting algorithm combines ideas from POMCP and message-passing approaches from Graphical Probabilistic Models.

The paper is structured as follows: First, we present relevant background material in Section 2. Then, in Section 3, we present the Graphical Partially Observable Markov Decision (GPOMDP) model and in Section 4 the Graphical Partially Observable Monte-Carlo Planning (GPOMCP) algorithm. The runtime behavior of the algorithm is evaluated based on a common benchmark scenario in Section 5. The paper concludes in Section 6 with a summary and future outlook.

2 Background

2.1 Partially Observable Markov Decision Problems

Markov Decision Processes (MDP) represent scenarios for decision-making under uncertainty where the system dynamics are dependent only on its current state and chosen actions, but not on the past history that lead to the current state [Put94]. Partially Observable Markov Decision Problems (POMDP) generalize MDP to situations where the underlying state is latent and can only be observed indirectly [KLC98]. Partially Observable Monte-Carlo Decision Problems (POMDP) are defined as n-tuples

$$\langle V = S \cup A \cup R \cup O, \{\mathcal{X}_v\}, P_S^0, P_S, P_O, R, T \rangle .$$

The variables $v \in V$ are made up of the latent-state S, actions A, rewards R and observations O. In every period $t \in \{1, \ldots, T\}$, they take on a value from a discrete domain in the state vector $\underline{x}^t \in \mathcal{X}_V = \times_{v \in V} \mathcal{X}_v$. For brevity, the components of the state vector are referred to as s^t, a^t, r^t and o^t. Alternatively, we index components with a subscript, e.g. $\underline{x}_J^t$ for some set $J \subseteq V$. The initial latent-state s^0 is drawn from the distribution P_S^0. Afterwards, at the beginning of every period t, the actions a^t are selected. The following latent-state, as well as the resulting rewards and observations are drawn according to

$$P_S(s^{t+1} \mid s^t, a^t), \quad r^t = R(s^t, a^t, s^{t+1}), \quad P_O(o^t \mid s^t, a^t, s^{t+1}) .$$

The latent-state variables are not known to the choice-making entity and only the history $h^t = (\mathcal{X}_A \times \mathcal{X}_R \times \mathcal{X}_O)^{t-1}$ of previous actions, rewards and observations can be used for action selection. Histories can be concatenated with values from the current period and the empty history is written as ϵ. A policy π is a deterministic mapping from the history of previous periods to current actions. Rewards are included in the history so that we may refer to them in algorithms that improve policies based on sampled scenario rollouts. But rewards are treated as unobservable for the policies themselves. The value of a policy is the expected reward over the T periods given by Bellman's equation. The goal of solving a POMDP is to find a policy of maximum value.

$$V_\pi^t(s^t, h^t) = \mathbb{E}\left[\sum_{\rho \in \underline{x}_R^t} \rho + \mathbb{1}_{t<T} V_\pi^{t+1}(s^{t+1}, h^t a^t r^t o^t) \,\middle|\, a^t = \pi(h^t)\right]$$

$$V(\pi) = \sum_{s \in \mathcal{X}_S} P_S^0(s) V_\pi^0(s, \epsilon)$$

The so-called Q-value is defined as the expected rewards for choosing action a after an observed history h and following the policy π afterwards.

$$Q_\pi^t(h^t, a^t) = \sum_{s^t} P(s^t \mid h^t)\, \mathbb{E}\left[\sum_{r \in r^t} r + \mathbb{1}_{t<T} V_\pi^{t+1}(s^t, h^t a^t r^t o^t)\right]$$

2.2 Monte-Carlo Tree Search and POMCP

Monte-Carlo Tree Search (MCTS) [BPW+12] is a recent approach to search for an optimal policy in multi-period scenarios. MCTS cyclically generates example rollouts and updates the estimation for the value of actions at a specific position in the scenario tree. If the scenario is deterministic, then the scenario tree has a branching factor according the number of possible action-choices in every period. If the scenario is stochastic, then the possible state-transitions lead to an additional branching. Algorithm 2.1 shows the generic MCTS algorithm with rollout for POMDP scenarios. The performance of MCTS largely depends on the selection of actions for exploration. The question is whether to select actions that have shown good performance in the past, or whether to analyze less-explored branches of the scenario tree that might contain some undiscovered potential. Recently, the Upper-Confidence Bound (UCB) princple originally developed for bandit-games [ACBF02] has become a popular choice. In UCB, actions are evaluated according to their past performance with an additional bias that favors actions for which less empirical evidence is available.

$$\widehat{Q}[ha] + \alpha \sqrt{\frac{\log(n[h])}{n[ha]}}$$

Algorithm 2.1 The Monte-Carl Tree Search Algorithm with rollout for POMDP

procedure MCTS
  INITIALIZE
  while enough time **do**
    $h \leftarrow$ ROLLOUT
    UPDATE(h)
  end while
  return BESTACTION
end procedure

procedure ROLLOUTPOMDP
  $h \leftarrow \epsilon$
  $s \sim P_S^0$
  for $t \in \{1, \ldots, T\}$ **do**
    $a \leftarrow$ EXPLORATIONACTION(h)
    $s' \sim P_S(s, a)$; $r \leftarrow R(s, a, s')$; $o \sim P_O(s, a, s')$
    $h \leftarrow haro$
    $s \leftarrow s'$
  end for
  return h
end procedure

Variables indexed with square brackets denote maps. The default value for any index is zero. The map $\widehat{Q}$ contains estimations of Q-values and is updated after every rollout. The counter n is increased by one every time a certain history occurs during the rollouts. The exploration/exploitation tradeoff can be tuned with the weighting parameter α. This leads to an exploration strategy that prunes less promising branches implicitly. Still, convergence is guarantueed for many algorithms employing UCB since every branch is visited infinitely often in the limit. UCB-based exploration has led to huge performance increases for many game-playing AIs, in particular those for games with large branching factors, such as Go [GKS$^+$12]. Partially Observable Monte-Carlo Planning (POMCP, [SV10]) is the application of UCB to solving POMDP in the MCTS framework (see Algorithm 2.2). Note that the value estimation update in POMCP is relatively simplistic. It just gives the average rewards experienced after a given history/action combination during the rollouts. This converges to the actual Q-value of optimal play since the UCB-based action selection will choose optimal actions infinitely more often in the limit. More complex update mechanisms, e.g. updating beliefs on the value of an action in a Bayesian setting, may lead to better estimations for a given set of samples. However, empirical evidence shows an advantage for algorithms with fast updates that process more rollout/update cycles for the same computational effort. Competitive implementations of POMCP process several hundred thousand rollouts per second.

Algorithm 2.2 The POMCP algorithm in the MCTS framework

procedure INITIALIZEPOMCP
> $n[\cdot] \leftarrow 0;\ \widehat{Q}[\cdot] \leftarrow 0$

end procedure

procedure UPDATEPOMCP(h)
> $\rho \leftarrow 0$
> **for** $t \in \{T, \dots, 1\}$ **do**
>> $\rho \leftarrow \rho + \sum_{r \in R} x_r^t$
>> $n[h^t] \leftarrow n[h^t] + 1$
>> $n[h^t a^t] \leftarrow n[h^t a^t] + 1$
>> $\widehat{Q}[h^t a^t] \leftarrow \widehat{Q}[h^t a^t] + \frac{\rho - \widehat{Q}[h^t a^t]}{n[h^t a^t]}$
>
> **end for**

end procedure

procedure EXPLORATIONACTIONPOMCP(h)
> **if** $\exists a : n[ha] = 0$ **then**
>> **return** $\sim U(\{a : n[ha] = 0\})$
>
> **end if**
> **return** $\arg\max_a \widehat{Q}[ha] + \alpha \sqrt{\frac{\log(n[h])}{n[ha]}}$

end procedure

procedure BESTACTIONPOMCP
> **return** $\arg\max_{a \in \mathcal{X}_A} \widehat{Q}[a]$

end procedure

2.3 Decentralized and Multiagent POMDP

Decentralized planning in POMDP settings requires superexponential time to solve in the worst case [BGIZ02]. Thus, recent work has focused on heuristic solvers and specific classes of Distributed POMDP where some underlying structure can be exploited. Examples for such models are ND-POMDP [NVTY05], Dec-POMDP [OSWV08] and I-POMDP [GD05]. Readers are referred to [SZ08] for an in-depth discussion and equivalence results. A comparison between Dec-POMDP, ND-POMDP and our approach GPOMDP is given at the end of the following section.

3 Graphical POMDP

Graphical POMDP (GPOMDP) are defined as n-tuples comprised of a standard POMDP with an additional set of agents I.

$$\langle V = S \cup A \cup R \cup O, \{\mathcal{X}_v\}, P_S^0, P_S, P_O, R, T, I \rangle .$$

Agents $I \in 2^V$ are choice-making entities. Every agent $i \subseteq V \setminus S$ has access to a subset of the actions $A_i = A \cap i$, rewards $R_i = R \cap i$ and observations $O_i = O \cap i$. Agents may overlap by sharing some variables $(i, j) \in I^2, \Delta_{ij} = i \cap j$. Overlapping agents are in the set of neighbours $N(i) = \{j \in I : \Delta_{ij} \neq \varnothing\}$. In distributed settings, variable sharing can be achieved via lossless communication of action choices and observations. Every agent i has access to a reduced history $h_i^t \in (\mathcal{X}_i)^{t-1}$ in time period t. The action-choices are made by either assigning disjoint controlled actions $A_i^C \subseteq A_i$ and local policies $\pi_i^t : (\mathcal{X}_i)^{t-1} \to \mathcal{X}_{A_i^C}$ to every agent or via some additional online coordination mechanism.

Relation to Dec-POMDP In Decentralized POMDP (Dec-POMDP) [BGIZ02], all action and observation variables are assigned to exactly one agent, so that $A = \times_i A_i$, $O = \times_i O_i$. Agents have access to their own actions and observations only. So all Dec-POMDP are GPOMDP, but GPOMDP are Dec-POMDP if and only if all agents are disjoint, i.e. $\forall (i, j) \in I^2, i \neq j \Rightarrow i \cap j = \varnothing$. However, it is possible to construct additional actions and observations in Dec-POMDP in a way that mimicks communication channels between agents [SZ08]. In consequence, for any given GPOMDP, a Dec-POMDP can be constructed that recovers sharing of actions via communication channels. Shared observations can be achieved by duplication of observation variables $P(x_{o'} \mid x_o) = \delta_{\{x_{o'} = x_o\}}$. This structure is however lost in the general Dec-POMDP and has to be rediscovered by the solvers.

Relation to ND-POMDP Networked Distributed POMDP (ND-POMDP) [NVTY05]) factorize the latent-state so that the variables are either controlled by exactly one agent or are unobservable $S = \times_i S_i \times S_u$. Action and observation variables are each assigned to a unique agent, so that $A = \times_i A_i$, $O = \times_i O_i$.

The agents are transition and observation independent and coupled only by the reward function.

$$P(s^{t+1} \mid s^t, a^t) = P(s_u^{t+1} \mid s_u^t) \prod_{i \in I} P(s_i^{t+1} \mid s_i^t, a_i^t)$$

$$P(o^t \mid s^t, a^t) = \prod_{i \in I} P(o_i^t \mid s_u^t, s_i^t, a_i^t)$$

$$R(s, a) = \sum_{c \in \mathcal{C}} R_c(u, s_c, a_c)$$

The reward function R in ND-POMDP is made up of components that depend on a cluster of agents $\mathcal{C} \in 2^I$. With a slight abuse of notation, the latent-state of a cluster is $s_c \in \times_{v \in \cup_c i} \mathcal{X}_v$ and similarle for actions. The resulting locality of interaction between agents is characterized by a graph $G_{\mathcal{C}} = (I, C := \{(i, j) \in I^2 : \exists c \in \mathcal{C}, i \in c, j \in c\})$. Most papers assuming the ND-POMDP model further allow agents to communicate observations with some or all the other agents. According to this definition, all ND-POMDP are GPOMDP. The reverse is not necessarily true, since GPOMDP do not impose transition and observation independence between agents.

4 Graphical POMCP

We now introduce the Graphical Partially Observable Monte-Carlo Planning (GPOMCP) algorithm for solving GPOMDP online in a distributed fashion. It draws from two main sources of inspiration: The POMCP algorithm [SV10], one of the state of the art online POMDP solvers, and message-passing approaches based on the Generalized Distributive Law (GDL) [AM00, KFL01]. Variants of the latter are known for example the Belief Propagation (BP) algorithm [Pea88] in Graphical Probabilistic Models and the Max-Plus algorithm used for Distributed Constraint Optimization (DCOP) [PF05].

Assume a GPOMDP where the agents form a hypergraph tree $H = (I, E)$ with agents as vertices and neighborhood relations as edges $E = \{(i, j) \in I^2 : j \in N(i)\}$. This assumption is motivated by BP, where convergence is also only guaranteed on trees. Still, BP on loopy graphs often achieves good results in practice [YFW+00]. The theoretical insight and empirical evidence to draw the analogy for GPOMCP is however not in the scope of this contribution. Since the visible actions A_i overlap, agents can select contradicting sets of actions. In Algorithm 4.1 this is resolved by giving precedence to agents who make their choice later. That is necessary, since the UCB-based action selection may otherwise lead to situations where two agents have each a strong preference for different but overlapping set of actions. Selecting a mixture of the two action sets can lead to a blocking situations where the same actions are selected indefinitely in a row as both agents were not able to see the action for which they have a strong preference. By giving precedence to later agents, at least one agent gets to see the results of his preferred action set and will eventually move on to a different choice.

Algorithm 4.1 Action selection in GPOMCP

procedure EXPLORATIONACTIONGPOMCP(h)
    $\underline{x}_A \in \mathcal{X}_A$
    for $i \in I$ **do**
        $\underline{y}_{A_i} \leftarrow$ AGENTEXPLORATIONACTIONGPOMCP(i, h_i)
        for $a \in A_i$ **do**
            $x_a \leftarrow y_a$
        end for
    end for
    return $\underline{x}_A$
end procedure
procedure AGENTEXPLORATIONACTIONGPOMCP(i, h_i)
    if $\exists a_i : n[h_i a_i] = 0$ **then**
        return $\sim U(\{a_i : n[h_i a_i] = 0\})$
    end if
    return $\arg\max_{a_i} \widehat{Q}_i[h_i a_i] + \alpha\sqrt{\frac{\log(n[h_i])}{n[h_i a_i]}}$
end procedure
procedure BESTACTIONGPOMCP(h)
    $\underline{x}_A \in \mathcal{X}_A$
    for $i \in I$ **do**
        $\underline{y}_{A_i} \leftarrow \arg\max_{a_i} \widehat{Q}_i[h_i a_i]$
        for $a \in A_i$ **do**
            $x_a \leftarrow y_a$
        end for
    end for
    return $\underline{x}_A$
end procedure

The update procedure of the POMCP algorithm consists of a message passing and an estimation update phase. The message passing phase uses a forward/backward schedule. Recall that the agents form a tree hyper-graph. The schedule $\mathcal{S}(I)$ contains an ordered list of sender/receiver relations where the agents i wait until they have received messages from their $|N(i)|-1$ children in the graph. Then they send out a messages to their parent. Once they have received a message from their parent, messages are sent out to all children. This is called the forward/backward schedule since the message exchange starts at the leaf of the tree, propagates through the graph and finally returns to the leafs. Note that the schedule can be efficiently implemented to run in parallel on distributed agents. But we omit discussing this possibility in this text.

Algorithm 4.2 Initialization and estimation update in GPOMCP

procedure INITIALIZEGPOMCP(I)
  $n[\cdot] \leftarrow 0$
  $\forall i \in I, \widehat{R}_i[\cdot] \leftarrow 0,\ \widehat{Q}_i[\cdot] \leftarrow 0$
  $\forall i \in I, \forall j \in N(i),\ n_{ij}[\cdot] \leftarrow 0,\ m_{i\to j}[\cdot] \leftarrow 0$
end procedure

procedure UPDATEGPOMCP(h)
  $\forall i \in I,\ \rho_i \leftarrow 0$
  $\forall i \in I, \forall j \in N(i),\ \rho_{ij} \leftarrow 0$
  for $t \in \{T, \ldots, 1\}$ **do**
    for $(i,j) \in \mathcal{S}(I)$ **do**
      $\rho_{ij} \leftarrow \rho_{ij} + \sum_{r \in (R\cap O_i)\setminus\Delta_{ij}} x_r^t$
      $n_{ij}[h_{ij}^t a_{ij}^t] \leftarrow n_{ij}[h_{ij}^t a_{ij}^t] + 1$
      $m_{i\to j}[h_{ij}^t a_{ij}^t] \leftarrow m_{i\to j}[h_{ij}^t a_{ij}^t] + \frac{\left(\rho_{ij} + \sum_{l\in N(i)\setminus j} m_{l\to i}[h_{il}^t a_{il}^t]\right) - m_{i\to j}[h_{ij}^t a_{ij}^t]}{n_{ij}[h_{ij}^t a_{ij}^t]}$
    end for
    for $i \in I$ **do**
      $\rho_i \leftarrow \rho_i + \sum_{r\in R\cap O_i} x_r^t$
      $n[h_i^t] \leftarrow n[h_i^t] + 1$
      $n[h_i^t a_i^t] \leftarrow n[h_i^t, a_i^t] + 1$
      $\widehat{R}_i[h_i^t a_i^t] \leftarrow \widehat{R}_i[h_i^t a_i^t] + \frac{\rho_i - \widehat{R}_i[h_i^t a_i^t]}{n[h_i^t a_i^t]}$
      $\widehat{Q}_i[h_i^t a_i^t] \leftarrow \widehat{R}_i[h_i^t a_i^t] + \sum_{j\in N(i)} m_{j\to i}[h_{ij}^t a_{ij}^t]$
    end for
  end for
end procedure

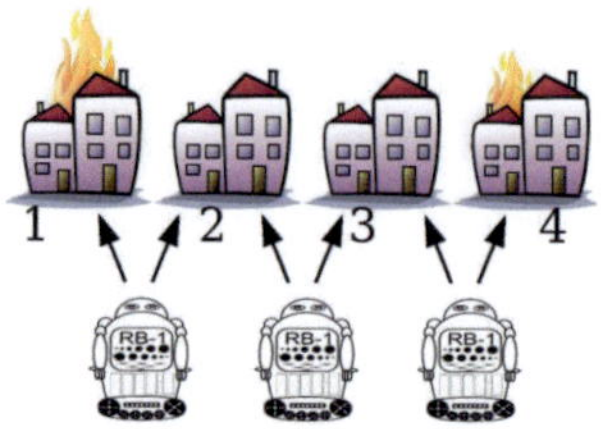

Figure 5.1: Illustration of the Firefighting benchmark problem taken from [OSWV08]

Similar to POMCP, the reward from the later periods is accumulated in a scalar ρ_i. However, ρ_i takes only the rewards into account that are visible to the agent i. In addition, we accumulate a set of summed rewards ρ_{ij} for every neighbour with the rewards that were visible to i, but not to the neigbhour $j \in N(i)$. The message from agent i to agent j then becomes an estimate for the amount of rewards the subtree behind the edge (i, j) is expected to receive during the current period and afterwards, conditioned on the joint history $h_{ij}^t \in (\mathcal{X}_{\Delta_{ij}})^t$ and action $a_{ij} \in \mathcal{X}_{A \cap \Delta_{ij}}$. The messages and the locally visible rewards are then used to update the local estimates for the true Q-Value.

5 Benchmark Results

We compare our results on the Firefighting domain introduced in [OSWV08]. It models a team of n firefighters that have to extinguish fires in a row of $n_H = n+1$ houses. In this work, we will take $n = 8$ and $T = 3$. Each house H has a fire level $l_H \in \{0, \ldots, 2\}$. The latent-state is an assignment of fire levels to every house. See Figure 5.1 for an illustration of the scenario.

At every time step, each firefighter f can choose to fight fires at house f or $f+1$. If a house H is burning ($l_H > 0$) and no firefighting agent is present, its fire level will increase by one point with probability 0.8 if any of its neighboring houses are burning, and with probability 0.4 if none of its neighbors are on fire. A house that is not burning can only catch fire with probability 0.8 if one of its neighbors is on fire. When two firefighters are at the same house, they will extinguish any present fire completely, setting the house's fire level to zero. A single agent present at a house will lower the fire level by one point with probability 1 if no neighbors are burning, and with probability 0.6 otherwise. Each firefighter can only observe whether there is a fire or not at its location. Fire is observed with probability 0.2 if $l_H = 0$, with probability 0.5 if $l_H = 1$, and with probability 0.8 otherwise. Rewards are $2 - l_H$ for each house according to the burn level reached in that period. Initially, the fire level l_H of each house is drawn from a uniform distribution. Each firefighter is represented by an agent that perceives the actions, rewards and observations of himself and of his neighbours $f - 1$ and $f + 1$ if they exist.

Figure 5.2 compares the performance of three approaches in the firefighting benchmark scenario. In all cases, we estimate Q-values with the given number of rollouts. Then, the resulting performance is evaluated as the mean reward of 500 rollouts where we choose the action with maximum estimated Q-value in every period. The first appraoch employs standard POMCP where all actions, rewards and observations are visible to a central learning an planning entity. The second approach is the FT-FV-MPOMDP algorithm from [AO15] where the first application of MCTS to Dec-POMDP in was given. The factored tree (FT) version of their algorithm is equal to GPOMCP when omitting the message passing step, therefore having each agent build up a separate evaluation. The last approach compared in the benchmark is our GPOMCP. All algorithms ran with an exploration weight factor of $\alpha = 10$.

The benchmark shows the results for running the rollout and update step for the given number of repetitions and then using the resulting Q-value estimates to guide the action selection during the T periods. Comparing the algorihtms in a pure online-planning scenario is planned for the near future.It can be seen that GPOMCP outperforms the other algorithms in the firefighting scenario. Both GPOMCP and FV-POMCP converge to a stable solution within 50,000 rollouts.

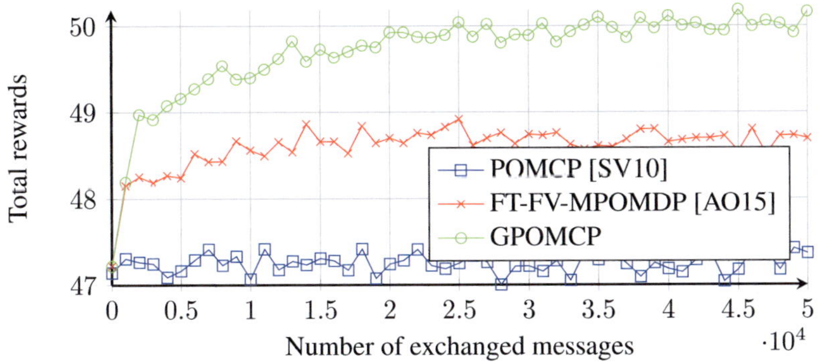

Figure 5.2: Benchmark results of the firefighting scenario.

However, GPOMCP achieves a substantially better solution. This is due to the coordination where agents also consider expected rewards even in parts of the POMDP that are not visible to them. The convergence of POMCP is even slower than what the graph indicates since POMCP has to iterate over all possible joint actions in every period. Since the number of joint actions grows exponentially in the number of action variables, the rollouts are computationally more expensive for POMCP.

6 Summary

In this contribution, we presented the Graphical Partially Observable Markov Decision Problem (GPOMDP) to capture the structure of Distributed POMDP where agents may overlap in their observable variables. Whe further introduced an algorithm for solving GPOMDP based on the well-known POMCP algorithm [SV10] and the message passing approach known from Graphical Probabilistic Models. First empirical evidence hints at favorable convergence properties for factorizable POMDP. Future work will apply GPOMCP to further benchmark problems from the literature and characterise its theoretical properties. Furthermore, we intend to apply GPOMCP to problems with continuous state and action spaces according to the principles developed in [BDMB13].

Bibliography

[ACBF02] Peter Auer, Nicolo Cesa-Bianchi, and Paul Fischer. Finite-time analysis of the multiarmed bandit problem. *Machine learning*, 47(2-3):235–256, 2002.

[AM00] Srinivas M Aji and Robert J McEliece. The generalized distributive law. *Information Theory, IEEE Transactions on*, 46(2):325–343, 2000.

[AO15] Christopher Amato and Frans A Oliehoek. Scalable Planning and Learning for Multiagent POMDPs. In *Twenty-Ninth AAAI Conference on Artificial Intelligence*, 2015.

[BDMB13] Lucian Busoniu, Andrew Daniels, Rémi Munos, and Robert Babuska. Optimistic planning for continuous-action deterministic systems. In *Adaptive Dynamic Programming And Reinforcement Learning (ADPRL), 2013 IEEE Symposium on*, pages 69–76. IEEE, 2013.

[BGIZ02] Daniel S Bernstein, Robert Givan, Neil Immerman, and Shlomo Zilberstein. The complexity of decentralized control of markov decision processes. *Mathematics of operations research*, 27(4):819–840, 2002.

[BPW+12] Cameron B Browne, Edward Powley, Daniel Whitehouse, Simon M Lucas, Peter I Cowling, Philipp Rohlfshagen, Stephen Tavener, Diego Perez, Spyridon

Samothrakis, and Simon Colton. A survey of monte carlo tree search methods. *Computational Intelligence and AI in Games, IEEE Transactions on*, 4(1):1–43, 2012.

[GD05] Piotr J Gmytrasiewicz and Prashant Doshi. A framework for sequential planning in multi-agent settings. *Journal of Artificial Intelligence Research*, pages 49–79, 2005.

[GKS+12] Sylvain Gelly, Levente Kocsis, Marc Schoenauer, Michele Sebag, David Silver, Csaba Szepesvári, and Olivier Teytaud. The grand challenge of computer go: Monte carlo tree search and extensions. *Communications of the ACM*, 55(3):106–113, 2012.

[KFL01] Frank R Kschischang, Brendan J Frey, and H-A Loeliger. Factor graphs and the sum-product algorithm. *Information Theory, IEEE Transactions on*, 47(2):498–519, 2001.

[KHL08] Hanna Kurniawati, David Hsu, and Wee Sun Lee. Sarsop: Efficient point-based pomdp planning by approximating optimally reachable belief spaces. In *Robotics: Science and Systems*, volume 2008. Zurich, Switzerland, 2008.

[KLC98] Leslie Pack Kaelbling, Michael L Littman, and Anthony R Cassandra. Planning and acting in partially observable stochastic domains. *Artificial intelligence*, 101(1):99–134, 1998.

[NVTY05] Ranjit Nair, Pradeep Varakantham, Milind Tambe, and Makoto Yokoo. Networked distributed pomdps: A synthesis of distributed constraint optimization and pomdps. In *AAAI*, volume 5, pages 133–139, 2005.

[OSWV08] Frans A Oliehoek, Matthijs TJ Spaan, Shimon Whiteson, and Nikos Vlassis. Exploiting locality of interaction in factored dec-pomdps. In *Proceedings of the 7th international joint conference on Autonomous agents and multiagent systems-Volume 1*, pages 517–524. International Foundation for Autonomous Agents and Multiagent Systems, 2008.

[Pea88] Judea Pearl. Probabilistic reasoning in intelligent systems: Networks of plausible inference. 1988.

[PF05] Adrian Petcu and Boi Faltings. DPOP: A Scalable Method for Multiagent Constraint Optimization. In *Proceedings of the International Joint Conferences on Artificial Intelligence (IJCAI)*, pages 266–271, 2005.

[Put94] Martin L Puterman. Markov decision processes: Discrete stochastic dynamic programming. 1994.

[SV10] David Silver and Joel Veness. Monte-carlo planning in large pomdps. In *Advances in neural information processing systems*, pages 2164–2172, 2010.

[SZ08] Sven Seuken and Shlomo Zilberstein. Formal models and algorithms for decentralized decision making under uncertainty. *Autonomous Agents and Multi-Agent Systems*, 17(2):190–250, 2008.

[YFW+00] Jonathan S Yedidia, William T Freeman, Yair Weiss, et al. Generalized belief propagation. In *NIPS*, volume 13, pages 689–695, 2000.

Surface Inspection Planning for Laser Line Scanners

Mahsa Mohammadikaji

Vision and Fusion Laboratory
Institute for Anthropomatics
Karlsruhe Institute of Technology (KIT), Germany
mahsa.mohammadikaji@kit.edu

Technical Report IES-2015-10

Abstract: The important role of automated visual methods in industrial product inspection necessitates the design of optimized and precise measurement setups. Due to the high dimensionality of the design space, the manual choice of the geometrical and optical parameters is tedious and often not optimal. In this article we study the problem of inspection planning for laser line scanners which are affordable and widely-used inspection tools. To this end, the measurement model is defined and appropriate evaluation metrics are introduced, which formulate the optimization problem in terms of a number of constrains and cost functions. Visibility analysis, lateral resolution, range resolution, and the measurement uncertainty are of the main metrics we cover. Computer graphics simulations are utilized to simulate the measurement in different setup configurations and estimate the evaluation metrics. We also propose a general uncertainty model which can be applied for modeling the uncertainty in laser scanners. The optimum laser scanner setup can be achieved by optimizing the defined evaluation metrics using a multi-objective approach.

1 Introduction

In the manufacturing process, an inspection is the process of determining if a product deviates from a set of given specifications [NJ95]. Depending on the product, different features can be of interest including completeness of the components, surface properties such as texture, and the geometrical dimensions. Based on the application, the desired geometrical features are also diverse. They can include 1D properties such as length, 2D profiles such as a circle, the 3D structure of the product, or other geometrical characteristics like flatness, cylindricity and parallelism. This report is mainly dedicated to the applications with the purpose of 3D geometrical inspection to acquire the spatial structure of the target product.

Depending on the application and the surface properties of the product as well as the allowed tolerances, different inspection techniques can be applied. Touch-trigger probes mounted on the coordinate measuring machines (CMMs) are a classical solution in industry. CMMs sample the product surface by touching it at specific points and provide micro-scale measurements [WPH06] with well-studied performance characteristics [ISO09], however, at a very low scan rate [NJ95]. In addition, the touch-probes are not applicable to deformable surfaces . Automated visual inspection methods (AVI), on the other hand, provide fast and contactless scanning of dense point-clouds, but typically achieve a lower accuracy [PLBR03]. Moreover, the performance of AVI methods can be affected by many environmental factors such as surface properties (*e.g.* reflectivity, roughness), illumination, and sensor calibration quality. These factors lead to an uncertainty in measurement whose analysis is rather complex [CBL02].

Due to the desired benefits that AVI methods provide, a precise setup design and planning is needed to optimize the acquisition and guarantee the measurement uncertainty. However, the design space for AVI setups are often very large. To this end, sensor planning methods have been developed to optimize the setups in terms of sensor view-points and optical parameters. Based on the application, a number of optimization criteria have been applied. Sensor visibility and optimum surface coverage are of the important issues frequently discussed in this context [Pit99]. A few planning methods have also included the measurement uncertainty metric into their optimization[PLBR03, Sco09].

In this report, we focus on the problem of CAD-based planning for laser line scanners, which are affordable and widely-used inspection tools based on the principle of triangulation [BLF15]. To discuss the issue, we have organized the main content of the article in five sections. Section 2 introduces the geometry and the measurement model of laser line scanners. We elaborate on the topic of inspection planning and discuss the different optimization criteria in section 3. The measurement uncertainty metric is particularly discussed and a proposed uncertainty modeling for laser line scanners is presented. Section 4 introduces our multi-objective approach for the optimization in brief. Finally, we conclude the discussion in section 5. Throughout this article, bold letters denote vectors and uppercase letters correspond to matrices.

2 Laser Line Scanners

Laser line scanners are a variant of structured-light scanners, in which a known illumination pattern is projection on the object and captured by a camera [BLF15]. In the case of laser line scanners, the structured light is a laser fan made by spreading the light of a laser beam through special lenses. Figure 2.1 illustrates the geometry of a laser line scanner. In this figure, the laser l emits a laser fan with an opening angle θ_l. This causes a 2D illuminated profile on the target surface which is captured by a camera located at $\mathbf{o_c}$. The received image is then processed to extract the intersection of the laser plane with the object surface with sub-pixel accuracy, using different peak detection algorithms [FN96].

The coordinate frame of the camera is spanned by the vectors $\mathbf{r}$, $\mathbf{u}$, and $\mathbf{v}$, and has a distance d_c with the world origin $\mathbf{o_w}$. The angle τ is referred to as the triangulation angle and θ_c is the angle between the camera axis and the horizon. During the inspection, the object is moved along the x-axis. The parameters d, θ_c and τ are important degrees of freedom in designing a laser scanner setup.

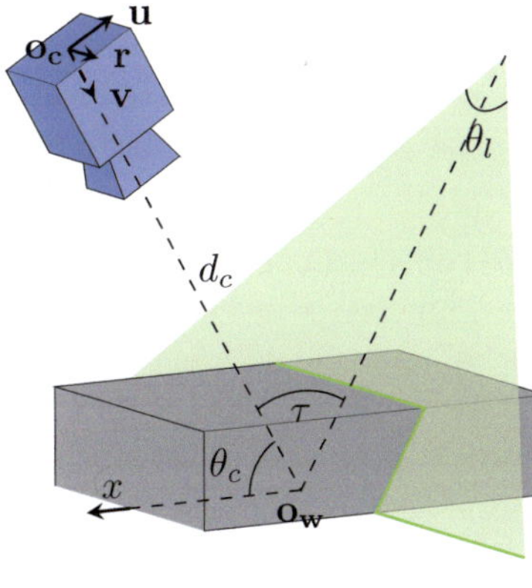

Figure 2.1: Geometry of a laser line scanner.

2.1 Measurement Model

The measurement model describes both the camera and the laser plane, as well as the way these models are connected to derive the 3D coordinates of a measurement point. In this section, we describe the parametrization and modeling of a laser scanner which is flexible to changing the setup parameters.

The camera projection is modeled by the well-known pin-hole camera model [MSKS12]. This model defines the relation between the world coordinates of a measurement point (x_w, y_w, z_w) and the 2D coordinates (x_p, y_p) of its projection on the image plane by:

$$\lambda \begin{bmatrix} x_p \\ y_p \\ 1 \end{bmatrix} = KP \begin{bmatrix} x_w \\ y_w \\ z_w \\ 1 \end{bmatrix} = \begin{bmatrix} f_x & s & c_x \\ 0 & f_y & c_y \\ 0 & 0 & 1 \end{bmatrix} \begin{bmatrix} R & \mathbf{t} \end{bmatrix} \begin{bmatrix} x_w \\ y_w \\ z_w \\ 1 \end{bmatrix}.$$

The projection matrix of a camera in this model is obtained by the multiplication of the matrix $K^{3\times 3}$, containing the intrinsic calibration parameters (f_x, f_y, s, c_x, c_y), and the matrix $P^{3\times 4}$, built by the concatenation of a 3D rotation matrix R, and a translation vector $\mathbf{t}$. In this equation, R and $\mathbf{t}$ determine the relative transformation of world to camera coordinate frame and λ is a scale factor. For simplicity, the skew parameter s is often considered to be zero.

The space illuminated by the laser is theoretically a part of a 3D plane. However in practice, the laser plane is obviously not infinitely thin, but rather it occupies a volume which depends on a number of factors including the lens used to spread the laser beam. Nevertheless, since the peak intensity at the lateral center of the illuminated profile is estimated and extracted on the image, we can still model the detected points as part of a 3D plane in space using

$$\mathbf{x}^{\mathrm{T}}\mathbf{n} = d, \tag{2.1}$$

in which $\mathbf{n}$ is the plane normal vector, $\mathbf{x} = \begin{bmatrix} x_w & y_w & z_w \end{bmatrix}^{\mathrm{T}}$ is a point in the world coordinate frame, and d is a scalar.

Equation (2.1) leads to two independent linear equations which are not enough to recover 3D coordinates. In the structured light scanning, the known structure of the emitted light serves as an additional information. In this case, the additional information is the laser plane equation, since the 2D detected points both fulfill the camera and laser plane equations. Therefore, by adding (2.1) to the two previously obtained equations, the system of linear equations

$$\begin{bmatrix} \mathbf{r}^{\mathrm{T}} - \mathbf{v}^{\mathrm{T}} \frac{(x_p - c_x)}{f_x} \\ \mathbf{u}^{\mathrm{T}} - \mathbf{v}^{\mathrm{T}} \frac{(y_p - c_y)}{f_y} \\ \mathbf{n}^{\mathrm{T}} \end{bmatrix} \begin{bmatrix} x_w \\ y_w \\ z_w \end{bmatrix} = \begin{bmatrix} \frac{(x_p - c_x)}{f_x} t_3 - t_1 \\ \frac{(y_p - c_y)}{f_y} t_3 - t_2 \\ d \end{bmatrix} \tag{2.2}$$

results, which is used to reconstruct the 2D detected points in the image. Vectors $\mathbf{r}^{\mathrm{T}}, \mathbf{u}^{\mathrm{T}}$, and $\mathbf{v}^{\mathrm{T}}$ (see Figure 2.1) are the row vectors of the rotation matrix or equivalently $R^{\mathrm{T}} = [\mathbf{r}\ \mathbf{u}\ \mathbf{v}]$, and t_i refers to an element of the translation vector $\mathbf{t} = [t_1\ t_2\ t_3]^{\mathrm{T}}$. To keep the notation concise, we use the expression $A\mathbf{x} = \mathbf{b}$ to refer to Eq. (2.2). Thus, to obtain the 3D measurement point $\mathbf{x}$, one can build matrix A and vector $\mathbf{b}$ accordingly and compute

$$\mathbf{x} = A^{-1}\mathbf{b}.$$

3 Evaluation Metrics in Sensor Planning

The possible design space for an AVI system is often very large. This includes the position and orientation of the camera(s) and illumination(s), and possibly the intrinsic camera parameters (*e.g.* focus, aperture). Therefore, manually selecting a configuration for this high-dimensional space is tedious and in most cases not optimal. Inspection planning seeks to automatically select a sensor configuration (or a sequence of them) which optimally fulfills some evaluation metrics. The majority of the works in this area is only devoted to optimizing the view-points of the sensors; however, a few authors have also included some optical constraints [Cow88] or the measurement uncertainty [MJR+11] in their planning.

The rest of this section is dedicated to introducing and reviewing the major optimization metrics which can potentially be used in view-point planning for designing 3D scanners. In addition, we point out our approach on how to include each metric in planning a laser line scanner.

3.1 Surface Coverage

The optimum surface coverage is of the main goals pursued in almost all planning methods. The aim is to select the sensor configurations automatically so as to cover the whole surface with a minimal number of acquisitions. This problem is equivalent to a set-cover problem in which finding the global optimum is known to be an NP-complete problem. Therefore, the approaches are usually greedy or approximate.

Based on the a priori available information, the methods with the purpose of full surface coverage fall into *model-based* and *non-model-based* categories [SRR03]. Non-model-based methods assume no a priori knowledge about the target object. This is usually the case when no CAD model is available, such as model acquisition of ancient statues or reverse engineering. An important variety of these methods are known as *next-best view planning* [Pit99], in which the next best view-point is the one that maximizes the information gain of the next measurement. Model-based methods, however, [Sco09] [PLBR03] base the planning on an a priori object model usually in the form of a CAD model. The view-point space is then discretized and the optimization is carried out in this space by means of different ray tracing algorithms to determine the visibility of each view-point and avoid occlusion.

Due to the availability of CAD models and the prior knowledge about the inspection work-space in industries, planning for industrial inspection purposes is typically model-based. Therefore, we also follow a model-based approach for the current application. To analyze the visibility based on a CAD model, one needs to determine the visibility of each surface primitive (e.g. mesh triangles) in every desired view-point. Based on the complexity of the model, the number of triangles in a model can be arbitrarily high. For instance, the CAD model of the cylinder head in Figure 3.1 contains more than 2 million triangles. Therefore, it is crucial that the visibility check for each triangle be efficient. To do so, we have implemented the *Rasterizing Simulation Library* (RSL) which is a hardware accelerated rendering tool based on *Open Graphics Library* (OpenGL). Figure 3.1 displays an image rendered by RSL which simulates the camera image during the inspection of a cylinder head. In each desired view-point, RSL enables us to determine the surface triangles which are seen by the camera and/or hit by the laser within milliseconds.

3.2 Lateral Resolution

Lateral resolution is a metric to evaluate the density of the scanned point-cloud based on the distance between adjacent 3D measured points. The sensor distance and the camera resolution are of the dominant factors influencing this metric. As the visibility metric prefers the view-points with a broader view, longer sensor distances are often preferred. Lateral resolution plays a complementary role in ensuring that the resulting point-cloud has the required resolution. Cowan

[Cow88] considers the lateral resolution as a constraint and proposes a simple estimation model based on the target distance and the camera pixel size. Scott [Sco09] has also proposed a model for a range scanner based on the distance, viewing angle and the image resolution.

For an arbitrary surface, the intersection of the laser on the surface can form an arbitrary curve whose scan resolution we want to estimate. During the simulation for the visibility analysis, we are able to obtain the true 3D points on the CAD model which are hit by the laser plane and projected on each column of the image. Therefore, the distance calculation for the adjacent 3D points in the resulting point-cloud is straightforward.

3.3 Range Resolution

Every measurement is assigned a resolution which indicates the smallest value that the measuring method is able to distinguish. For a laser line scanner, the range resolution can be defined as the minimum change of the target height which can be distinguished by the sensor. To determine the range resolution one needs to determine the change in the surface height which induces the minimum allowed change in the position of the laser line on the image, which is in turn equal to the precision of the peak detection algorithm.

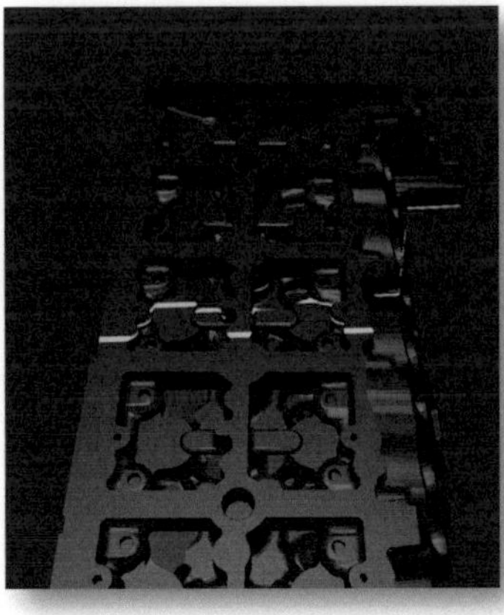

Figure 3.1: Rendering an image from the camera view using RSL.

The sensitivity of laser scanners typically increases as the triangulation angle is increased in the interval $(0, \pi)$ [BLF15]. This fact can be utilized as a priority for the sensor view-point during the planning. To the best of our knowledge, range resolution has not yet been considered in the previous planning methods.

3.4 Measurement Uncertainty

Every measurement is subject to some level of uncertainty. According to the *Guide to the Expression of Uncertainty in Measurement (GUM)* [JCG08], every measurement needs to be accompanied with a statement about its uncertainty so that one is able to assess the measurement reliability. An uncertainty is expressed in terms of a standard deviation (for a single measurement) or a covariance matrix (for multi-variable measurements such as the 3D coordinates) which describes the dispersion of the measurement around the mean value.

Methodologies to evaluate the measurement uncertainty are generally categorized into two types. Type A methods are based on the calculation of sample mean and variance of repeated measurements. Type B methods on the other hand, rely on a scientific judgment based on all of the available information on the possible variability of the measurement. This is often done by propagating the input uncertainties through the measurement model. Despite of the standard uncertainty evaluation methods, the inclusion of the uncertainty metric in the sensor planning is not straightforward since one needs an uncertainty model that thoroughly describes the measurement uncertainty in each configuration.

In the rest of this section, we review and analyze the methodologies for estimating and modeling the uncertainty. In Section 3.4.3, we introduce our approach towards modeling the uncertainty of a laser line scanner.

3.4.1 Type A Uncertainty Evaluation Methods

The methods following a type A uncertainty evaluation typically include a large amount of experimental work and the measurement uncertainty is estimated by analyzing repeated measurements in different configurations. Most of the previous works in modeling the uncertainty of laser scanners belong to the type A category.

The experimental uncertainty model used by Scott [Sco09] is experimentally obtained during the calibration. This model grows quadratically with the distance and has an inverse cosine relation with the incident angle. Prieto et al. [PLBR03] suggest an empirical model depending quadratically on the distance and exponentially on the orientation angles of the sensor. The uncertainty model proposed by Mahmud et al. [MJR$^+$11] depends only on the laser beam incidence angle. Contri et al. [CBL02] experimentally analyze the uncertainty of reference point detection during the calibration, which is further propagated to the reconstruction of the points using type B methods.

Since the inaccuracies in the detection of the laser line on the image highly depend on the surface reflection and micro-structure, the laser detection process is an important source of uncertainty. The previously mentioned works depend on reference objects to analyze the error and therefore, their models are biased by the surface properties of the reference objects and the quality of their calibration. Moreover, the differences in their resulting models indicate that one cannot make a general statement about the behavior of the sensor uncertainty and therefore, the experiments need to be repeated for every individual sensor.

3.4.2 Type B Uncertainty Evaluation Methods

Type B analysis is often used to propagate the estimated input uncertainties to the output measurement. Clarke [Cla98] presents two alternatives for modeling and propagation of uncertainties: Monte-Carlo simulation and first order error propagation, which we review below. We also discuss about a third alternative with a non-probabilistic approach.

Monte Carlo Simulations are based on the repeated sampling of the input random variables according to their probability distribution, to estimate the probability distribution of the output measurement. This method has a low implementation overhead and can be applied to all types of distributions [Cla98]; however, the sampling space grows exponentially with the input dimension which slows down the run-time as the number of uncertainty parameters increase. Using Monte Carlo simulations for sensor planning implies that the process should be repeated in each constellation and for every measurement point, which is not feasible. However, it can be utilized to evaluate the validity of other approximate methods.

Taylor-Based Uncertainty Propagation methods rely on direct mathematical propagation of the covariance matrix of the sources of uncertainty through the Taylor series expansion of the measurement function. Since the covariance propagation through nonlinear functions is cumbersome, these methods are most often based on a linear approximation, which can be valid as long as the input uncertainties are small. The method leads to a closed form mathematical expression which can be evaluated efficiently for each desired set of model parameters.

However, the approximation is less valid for highly nonlinear measurement models and large input uncertainties. In this approach, both input and output variables are typically considered to be Gaussian.

The measurement covariance matrix Σ_y obtained by a first-order approximation is given by

$$\Sigma_y = \boldsymbol{J_f} \Sigma_x \boldsymbol{J_f}^{\mathrm{T}}.$$

In this equation, $\mathbf{y} = f(\mathbf{x})$ is the measurement function, Σ_x is the covariance matrix of the input $\mathbf{x}$, and the Jacobian matrix of the measurement function is denoted by $\mathbf{J_f} = \frac{\partial f}{\partial \mathbf{x}}$.

Non-probabilistic methods typically assume fixed intervals to bound the dispersion of each input variable. Interval analysis methods, for example, use interval arithmetic operations [AM00]. The intervals are further propagated through the model to obtain the resulting measurement interval. However, the arithmetic operations are typically limited to a set of basic operations. These methods do not have a probabilistic point of view and are more adequate for worst-case system analysis. Nevertheless, by replacing the probability distributions with intervals, these methods relieve the assumption of Gaussian distributions. Telle et al. [TSY+05] have followed an interval analysis approach to propagate the uncertainties through a stereo visual system.

3.4.3 Proposed Uncertainty Modeling

In this section, we propose an uncertainty modeling for a laser line scanner, which can be used as one of the evaluation functions in sensor planning. Our intention is to present a general model where most of the differences in various setups (*e.g.* target object properties, sensor parameters, different calibration methods and positioning devices) can be addressed.

The prerequisite of an uncertainty modeling is the correct recognition and modeling of the sources of uncertainty. Since the sources can be numerous, it is tedious or even impossible to model every single factor. Every source of uncertainty, regardless of its properties, can eventually influence the resulting measurement by perturbing either of the parameters in the measurement model. Therefore, our approach is to model the effect of the uncertainty factors, rather than modeling the factors themselves. With all the sources of uncertainty taken into account, the error-free equation of the form $A\mathbf{x} = \mathbf{b}$ (see Section 2.1) will be replaced by the perturbed form:

$$(A + \delta A)(\mathbf{x} + \boldsymbol{\delta x}) = (\mathbf{b} + \boldsymbol{\delta b}).$$

The first step is the modeling and estimation of input uncertainties δA and $\delta \mathbf{b}$. By propagating the uncertainty using a type B method, the resulting measurement uncertainty $\delta \mathbf{x}$ can be obtained. To model the input uncertainties, we group the input parameters based on the part of the measurement they influence. This approach simplifies the incorporation of the numerous influencing factors and helps explain the differences in the previous models [Sco09, PLBR03]. We model the uncertainties in three categories which we briefly describe below:

Laser Detection Uncertainty: The inaccuracies in the detection of the 2D coordinates $\{x_p, y_p\}$ of the laser line on each column of the image are modeled by Gaussian additive noise parameters $\{x_p + e_{x_p}, y_p + e_{y_p}\}$. This uncertainty can be caused by several factors such as surface properties, laser speckle, sensor noise, quantization effects, and the sub-pixel peak detection algorithm. This model can be used to incorporate the target surface effect in the uncertainty model.

Positioning Uncertainty: Positioning devices are subject to some level of geometrical uncertainties in positioning the sensor. We model the geometrical uncertainties of the camera and laser independently, so as to allow a high degree of freedom in the view-planning. As shown in Figure 3.2, the positioning uncertainties lead to a transformation of the camera coordinate frame by a vector $\mathbf{e}_o$ and some rotation matrix R_e, both modeled as multivariate Gaussian distributions. The position and orientation of the laser plane is also affected by geometrical uncertainties. The deviations of the laser plane normal vector is modeled by a cone

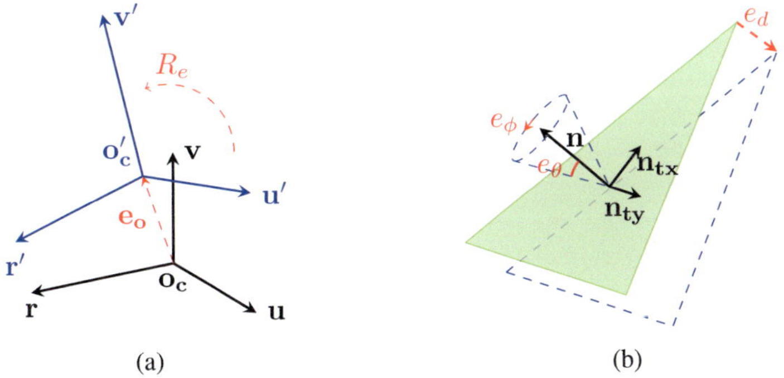

Figure 3.2: Positioning uncertainty models for camera coordinate frame (a) and laser plane (b).

parameterized by two independent random variables e_θ and e_ϕ. The random variable e_θ is considered to be a Gaussian variable and e_ϕ is uniformly distributed on the interval $[-\pi, \pi]$.

Intrinsic Calibration Uncertainty: The process of camera calibration is an important source of uncertainty. We assume that the camera model has no systematic bias and the variance and covariance of the uncertainties involved with the camera model parameters are extracted during the calibration using methods such as the one proposed by Leo and Paolillo [DP11]. Using such methods, the uncertainties in the intrinsic camera parameters can be modeled and integrated to the sensor uncertainty model.

Based on the uncertainty modeling discussed above, each original measurement parameter is perturbed by a number of random variables. Therefore, we can augment the measurement model by replacing each parameter with its perturbed form. By doing so, the augmented measurement model will be defined by the original parameters as well as the random variables describing the uncertainties. Using appropriate type B methods (*e.g.* first-order propagation), one can propagate the uncertainties of the random variables through the measurement model and estimate the covariance matrix of the resulting 3D measurement. This leads to a mathematical expression which can be evaluated for each measurement point and each desired setup constellation.

4 Optimization Approach

We carry out the optimization by searching in the discretized parameter space. The parameters of interest mainly include the camera position, orientation, and the triangulation angle, which together define a constellation. We use a multi-objective optimization approach, in which we try to find the optimum configuration of the laser and the camera according to the different metrics discussed in Section 3. The minimum required lateral resolution and range resolution are formulated in terms of optimization constraints. The measurement uncertainty and visibility metrics are the main optimization cost functions which need to be optimized by taking the constraints into account. Using RSL, the measurable surface points in each constellation can be extracted. The simulated point-cloud can be used to evaluate the visibility and the lateral resolution. The range resolution can also be judged according to the constellation parameters. Using the proposed uncertainty modeling and a first-order uncertainty propagation, the measurement uncertainty can be propagated to the simulated measurement points to obtain a covariance matrix. The covariance matrix describes the point's 3D dispersion ellipse, which can be used to evaluate the dispersion along any direction of interest by a linear transformation. The uncertainty along the surface normal is a good metric to evaluate the deviation of the measurement from the nominal surface. By computing all the needed metrics, the optimum setup design parameters can be found in a multi-objective optimization.

5 Conclusion

In this report, we studied the problem of setup design and optimization for laser line scanners. We first introduced the mathematical measurement model which maps a 2D detected point in the image to a 3D measurement point. We further studied different evaluation metrics, namely the visibility, lateral resolution, range resolution, and measurement uncertainty, which can be utilized to evaluate the setup from different evaluation perspectives. To analyze the visibility and the lateral resolution, the Rasterizing Simulation Library (RSL) was introduced which is used to render images from the camera view. An uncertainty model was also proposed in which appropriate random variables model the sources of uncertainty. By propagating the uncertainties, the induced uncertainty in the resulting 3D measurement can be estimated and expressed in terms of a covariance matrix. We finally discussed the optimization approach where we take all the evaluation metrics into account and optimize the setup in a multi-objective optimization.

6 Acknowledgments

We would like to kindly acknowledge Mr. Stephan Bergmann from the Computer Graphics Group at the Karlsruhe Institute of Technology for the development of the graphical simulations. Our further regards go to Mr. Stephan Irgendfried from the Intelligent Process Control and Robotics Lab (IPR) at Karlsruhe Institute of Technology for his support and cooperation in the project.

Bibliography

[AM00] Götz Alefeld and Günter Mayer. Interval analysis: theory and applications. *Journal of computational and applied mathematics*, 121(1):421–464, 2000.

[BLF15] Jürgen Beyerer, Fernando Puente León, and Christian Frese. *Machine Vision: Automated Visual Inspection: Theory, Practice and Applications*. Springer, 2015.

[CBL02] A. Contri, P. Bourdet, and C. Lartigue. Quality of 3d digitised points obtained with non-contact optical sensors. *CIRP Annals - Manufacturing Technology*, 51(1):443–446, 2002.

[Cla98] John C. Clarke. Modelling uncertainty: A primer. *University of Oxford. Dept. Engineering science, Tech. Rep*, 2161:98, 1998.

[Cow88] C. K. Cowan. Model-based synthesis of sensor location. In *Proceedings. 1988 IEEE International Conference on Robotics and Automation*, pages 900–905, 24-29 April 1988.

[DP11] G. Di Leo and A. Paolillo. Uncertainty evaluation of camera model parameters. In *2011 IEEE International Instrumentation and Measurement Technology Conference (I2MTC)*, 2011.

[FN96] R. B. Fisher and D. K. Naidu. A comparison of algorithms for subpixel peak detection. In Jorge L. C. Sanz, editor, *Image Technology*, pages 385–404. Springer Berlin Heidelberg, Berlin, Heidelberg, 1996.

[ISO09] Geometrical product specifications (GPS)–Acceptance and reverification tests for coordinate measuring machines (CMM)–Part 2: CMMs used for measuring linear dimensions. ISO 10360-2:2009, 2009.

[JCG08] Evaluation of Measurement data–Guide to the Expression of Uncertainty in Measurement. JCGM 100:2008, 2008.

[MJR+11] Mussa Mahmud, David Joannic, Michaël Roy, Ahmed Isheil, and Jean-François Fontaine. 3d part inspection path planning of a laser scanner with control on the uncertainty. *Computer-Aided Design*, 43(4):345–355, 2011.

[MSKS12] Yi Ma, Stefano Soatto, Jana Kosecka, and S Shankar Sastry. *An invitation to 3-d vision: from images to geometric models*, volume 26. Springer Science & Business Media, 2012.

[NJ95] Timothy S. Newman and Anil K. Jain. A survey of automated visual inspection. *Computer Vision and Image Understanding*, 61(2):231–262, 1995.

[Pit99] Richard Pito. A solution to the next best view problem for automated surface acquisition. *Pattern Analysis and Machine Intelligence, IEEE Transactions on*, 21(10):1016–1030, 1999.

[PLBR03] Flavio Prieto, Richard Lepage, Pierre Boulanger, and Tanneguy Redarce. A cad-based 3d data acquisition strategy for inspection. *Machine Vision and Applications*, 15(2):76–91, 2003.

[Sco09] William R. Scott. Model-based view planning. *Machine Vision and Applications*, 20(1):47–69, 2009.

[SRR03] William R. Scott, Gerhard Roth, and Jean-François Rivest. View planning for automated three-dimensional object reconstruction and inspection. *ACM Computing Surveys*, 35(1):64–96, 2003.

[TSY+05] B. Telle, O. Stasse, K. Yokoi, T. Ueshiba, and F. Tomita. Three characterizations of 3d reconstruction uncertainty with bounded error. In *2005 IEEE International Conference on Robotics and Automation*, pages 3894–3899, 18-22 April 2005.

[WPH06] A Weckenmann, G Peggs, and J Hoffmann. Probing systems for dimensional micro-and nano-metrology. *Measurement Science and Technology*, 17(3):504, 2006.

Algorithms and ideas on measuring 3D particles with cost efficient hardware

Peter Frühberger

Vision and Fusion Laboratory
Institute for Anthropomatics
Karlsruhe Institute of Technology (KIT), Germany
peter.fruehberger@kit.de

Technical Report IES-2015-11

Abstract: Measuring the volume of dirt particles within the context of technical cleanliness is an important task. The estimated 3D shape yields significant information about material properties and can highlight potential risks while using the produced goods within the final product. The results of this analysis are used to optimize the production steps to eliminate such harmfully shaped particles already in the early stages. Estimating 3D volume of particles with just a few microns of surface area normally implies an expensive microscope measuring device. This report investigates on hardware and software approaches to implement a cost efficient sensor consisting of standard components. A hardware setup using eight LED lights for illuminating the specimen from various known directions while using the shadow casts to reconstruct the object surface are proposed and evaluated. By manipulating the intensity of these LEDs the setup can be adjusted to be useful for various specimen with different reflection properties. The height of a particle is estimated at discrete positions based on a global model. Measurement results acquired by established state-of-the-art microscopes are analyzed for incorporation into the donated model for initial ground-truth. During the calibration process those results are used to map measured height values to the scalar z-values used for height estimation of the given specimen.

1 Introduction

Technical cleanliness is used to document and identify contamination on produced parts and surfaces. Quality assurance in other applications is directly applied on the examined object with optical or tactile measurement devices like camera systems, light-microscopy and interferometry. In technical cleanliness this approach is not feasible, because the particles of interest are not visible from the outside. Engine blocks, tubes and closed housings need special constructions and automation solutions in order to examine these goods with given measurement sensors directly. Therefore an intermediate step for extracting the particles out of the specimen (extraction) is introduced [dA14]. The part is washed with e.g. demineralized or alcohol assorted water and the outflow is filtered. The contamination in form of dirt particles is examined with given inspection devices after this extraction. Depending on the optical contrast conditions, filter material and dirt particle properties, the filter needs to be dried in a further post-processing step. Figure 1.1 is illustrating where the initial extraction process takes place.

There are different particles to be measured as shown in Figure 1.1. This non complete selection of different particle-types outlines several problems. Threads as seen in Figure 1.2(c) need to be unwrapped and their length needs to be estimated. Because of the extraction process, particles might conglomerate. This puts high demands on the software algorithms to segment the particle from the background and to segment the particles from each other 1.2(b). In this report we concentrate on single particles, well separated from the background by using established segmentation methods, as we are interested in finding an estimation of particle's height. Though the lateral dimensions are also relevant as the shape of the particle is needed to segment it from the background.

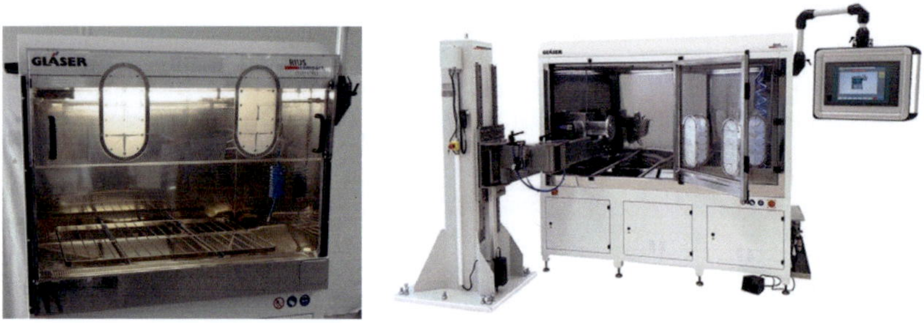

(a) (b)

Figure 1.1: In the extraction step dirt particles are washed out of the examined technical good (a). A complete cleaning setup can be seen in (b). Images source: Gläser Company (Horb).

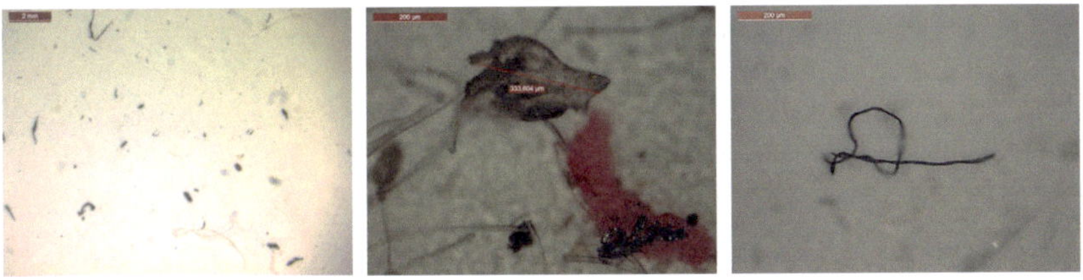

(a) (b) (c)

Figure 1.2: An overview acquired with a Leica Z-16 microscope is shown on (a). A detailed view of a conglomerate of particles in (b). It is further mandatory to unwrap eventual threads as seen in (c).

Estimating volume and 3D shape of dirt particles in the context of technical cleanliness is a crucial task as it yields important information concerning the risks such particles might cause inside technical components. [dA14] defines particles within a range of 50 to 1000 μm diameter as mandatory to be detectable. The inspection system therefore needs to provide a sufficient acquisition resolution and suitable optical properties like depth of focus in combination with a movable z-axis to reconstruct height information as shown in [FKB14]. A typical particle filter has a diameter of around 7 cm, which makes a moving table mandatory when examining the complete filter. Though estimation of 3D shape and volume is not yet a mandatory specification demanded by the standards [dA14], it is quite clear that the impact of harmful shaped particles occurring as conglomerations emerged by accumulations in the use-case scenario is quite considerable. Because of this reason 3D shape measurement and volume estimation was added into the appendix of the above specification and is likely to be mandatory in upcoming revisions.

This technical report describes an image processing approach in combination with a developed hardware illumination for detecting and analyzing clotted residuals on particle filters after the initial extraction and drying process as seen in figure 1.2. Those ideas were summarized and presented at the 3rd International Multidisciplinary Microscopy and Microanalysis Conference in October 2015 [FSB16]. This report at hand extends these results and examines the robustness of the described approach. It also presents errors in the volume estimation when shadow detection fails through misinterpretation of contours or noise in the acquired image. It formulates ideas to limit regions with suitable shadow per particle out of given geometry.

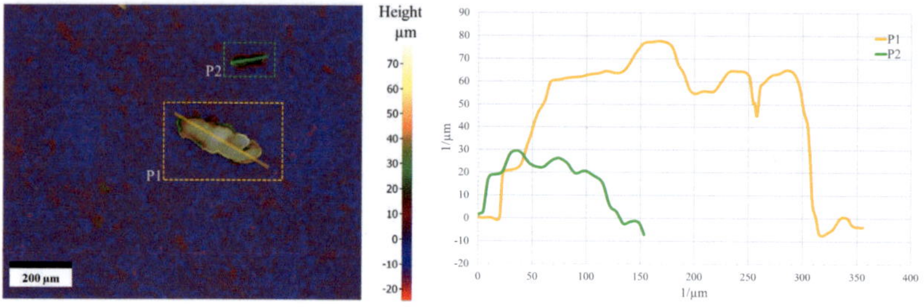

(a) (b)

Figure 1.3: Alicona InfinitFocus reconstruction of the lateral area shown as 2.5D (a) and the corresponding profile of the selected particles (b).

Figure 1.3 is showing a randomly selected particle filter analyzed with an Alicona InfinitFocus microscope. It can be seen, that estimating height information is a demanding task even for specialized measurement devices. The height of one of the particles seen in 1.3(a) is around 20 μm. Imitating professional measurement devices by replicating such a depth from focus setup is not feasible from a cost-efficient point of view, as accurate, e.g. a few microns moving z-axis within a low uncertainty level are expensive. Furthermore the optical lenses needed would be counterproductive against the need to examine a rather large lateral area.

1.1 Experimental setup and software implementation

The experimental setup consists of three components, a custom-built double LED ring light in combination with an industrial camera equipped with a bi-telecentric objective lens. The LEDs used in this setup are fabricated by Nichia company having a color temperature of 5000 K while providing 4.16 W electrical power. The angle of radiation is specified as 120° and therefore suitable for uniform illumination. Based on experimental results those LEDs are also suitable to produce sharp shadows, which is the most important criterion when segmenting the shadow contours from the background. The illumination is a combination of two separate rings, the lowermost ring consists of eight LEDs arranged equally spaced to illuminate the specimen from a flat angle as shown in Figure 1.4(c).

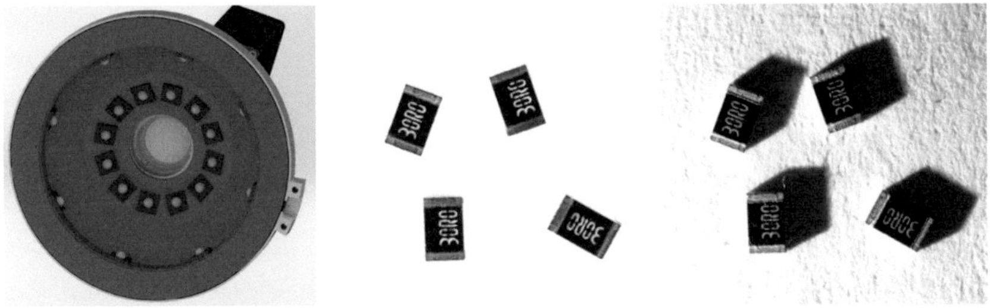

(a) Ringlight with LED rings (b) Overview image (c) Shadow demonstration

Figure 1.4: The illumination ring consists of two separately controllable LED rings (a). It can be used for uniformly illuminated overview images (b), while the lower ring produces sharp shadows (c).

This ring is used for generating the shadow contours. An upper ring is utilized to acquire homogeneous illuminated overview images (Figure 1.4(b)).

The second component is an industrial color camera Manta G-419C of ALLIED Vision Technologies with a resolution of 2048 × 2048 pixels. In our experiments the color sensor is not used. Segmentation and shadow detection is computed on the gray-scale image only. This camera was combined with the bi-telecentric objective TC 2M HR 016-C manufactured by Opto Engineering. The setup allows a pixel size of 4.5 $\mu\mathrm{m}^2$ and a depth of view of 2.0 mm. Therefore the field of view is $9.2 \times 9.2\ \mathrm{mm}^2$. In order to scan larger surfaces, this setup can be extended with a motorized stage as shown in [FSB15]. The software implementation, which consists of the shadow detection, calibration and 3D estimation, was realized in C++ using the opencv image processing library [Bra00].

2 Algorithm and implementation

Essential to the 3D reconstruction is a robust calibration. In the initial algorithm step an estimation of the light positions $\boldsymbol{L}_i$ in three-dimensional space is computed. Our coordinate-system fixates the center point $\boldsymbol{p_c} = \left(c_x,\ c_y,\ z\right)^T$ of the spanned vector space $\mathbf{0}$ at the center of the projected image scene. The unit of this vector is *pixel* in the x and y dimension. The z dimension is a scalar value mapped to a metric scale by comparing to ground-truth height measurements or a-priori known height measurement of a common specimen, acquired with a standardized microscope. We furthermore assume a punctual light source $\boldsymbol{L}_i$ and a list of correspondences $C_i = \{c_{jk}\}$ with $|C_i| \geq 2$, c_{jk} representing a point on the object $\boldsymbol{o_j}$ and a corresponding shadow contour point $\boldsymbol{s_k}$. It is possible to construct equations of lines $l(c_{jk})$ with $\boldsymbol{o_j}$ as support vector and $t \cdot (\boldsymbol{s_k} - \boldsymbol{o_j})$ with $t \in \mathbb{R}$ as the direction vector. The light source $\boldsymbol{L}_i$ can then be estimated by finding the intersection points by pairwise constructing lines $l(c_{jk})$ and $l(c_{j'k'}), j' \neq j, k' \neq k$. Because of deviations when computing the corresponding points a single intersection point might not necessarily exist. Therefore the problem is solved by finding the point $\boldsymbol{p}$ with minimal euclidean distance to all given lines out of C_i, donated as $dist(\boldsymbol{p}, l)$ to yield an estimation for $\boldsymbol{L_i}$. In a next iteration to this optimization problem outliers, lines that increase the variance of the distance deviation, can be filtered out to compensate incorrectly mapped correspondences. The non weighted optimization problem, where every correspondence has the same influence on the estimation position of $\boldsymbol{L_i}$ is provided as follows:

$$\boldsymbol{L}_i = \arg\min_{\boldsymbol{p}} \sum_{\substack{j,k \\ j \neq k}} dist(\boldsymbol{p}, l(c_{jk}))$$

An example correspondence mapping is shown in Figure 2.1(a). The calibration needs to be estimated for all LEDs in the given setup. To find the correspondence points, knowledge of the light source's position can be incorporated. It is helpful to choose simple specimens for calibration. In our example the corresponding points could be estimated by using a Harris corner detector as shown in [BPLF12] and [GW08]. In combination with the overview image Figure 1.4(b) corner candidates located on the object and others introduced by shadow can be distinguished as those appear in both images. False positives can be eliminated by taking previously known symmetric constraints into account. As the calibration is a crucial part concerning the accuracy of this method a manual calibration, implemented as a wizard in software is highly recommended. Figure 2.1(b) illustrates the algorithm for determining the height value at different positions (red circles) on the image plane. The outer contour of a shadow area S_i introduced by LED $\boldsymbol{L}_i$ can be estimated by masking the segmented specimen itself with the post-processed overview image Figure 2.2(b). After applying a threshold to segment the shadow from the background the contour can be estimated by computing its outline with morphological operators and edge detection. As we are only interested in those parts of the outer boundary, that have at least a minimum

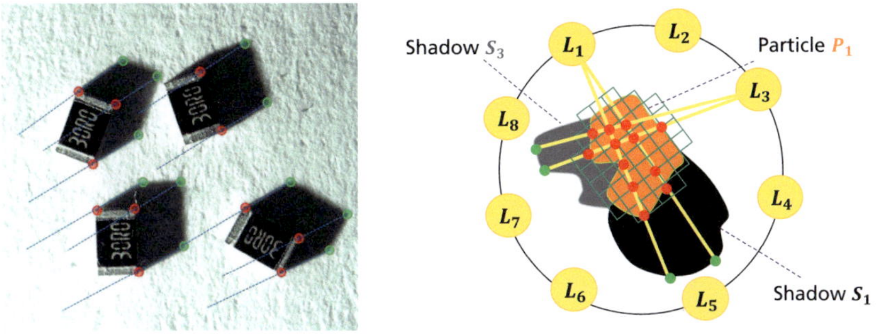

(a) Ringlight (b) overviewlights

Figure 2.1: Correspondences object (red) and shadow points (green) are maintained in a correspondence list C_i (a). The height at every position on the object is iteratively estimated through LED $\boldsymbol{L_i}$ and shadow boundary points B_i by finding the minimum z-value (b).

distance from the specimen itself in the direction of light position, those non relevant candidates are removed by multiplying the contour image with a slightly enlarged mask. The result can be seen in Figure 2.2(a). With the position of $\boldsymbol{L}_i$ and the shadow boundary points $B_i = \{s_0, \ldots, s_n\}$, containing all shadow points s_n produced by the light source out of the direction $\boldsymbol{L}_i$, a height value can be assigned to every pixel position $\boldsymbol{q} = \left(x,\, y,\, 0\right)^T$ on the image plane. The height value is computed by an orthogonal projection of the lines of sight $l_{ii}(\boldsymbol{L}_i, B_i)$ between the LED $\boldsymbol{L}_i$ and all corresponding shadow boundary points B_i as shown in Figure2.1(b). This procedure is repeated for all calibrated LEDs in this setup. While computing the height values produced by a single light-source $\boldsymbol{L_i}$ a maximum rule is assumed, which means that a larger height value is kept. This cares for artifacts introduced by the assumption of a point light source, which would produce borders of the specimen with a height h of zero, because the shadow path starts right next to the edge of the specimen. This maximum rule is only applied if there was no better height, e.g. lower height assigned by another light-source $\boldsymbol{L_j}$. That means, height values assigned by the computation of a different light-source are evaluated by maintaining a minimum rule. The height value h' at position $\boldsymbol{q'}$ is therefore only updated whenever the new height value is lower than the current value, which assigned by different light-source. The algorithm iterates over all light-sources, starting with on randomly selected light. The order does not matter, but every light and corresponding shadow points are only evaluated once. The line is constructed from the direction of the light-source and ends on the particle filter with height $z = 0$. After the iteration is finished the mask computed in a prior step multiplied by the image to eliminate artifacts located outside of the object.

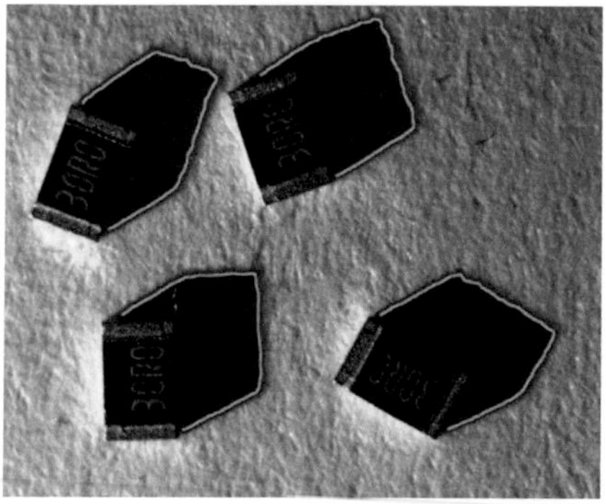

(a)

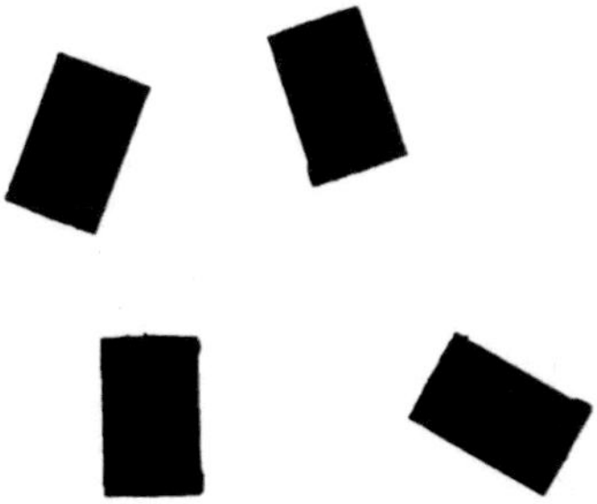

(b)

Figure 2.2: Outline is extracted by image processing algorithms (a). A mask is computed for later segmentation of the resulting height estimation (b).

3 Results

When directly comparing the results with measurements acquired by a professional system as illustrated in Figure 3.1(a) one can directly see that the height resolution of the microscope is much higher than the reconstruction seen in Figure 3.1(b) and 3.1(c). The microscope reconstructs the surface in much greater detail, taking properties of the surface like roughness into account. As seen on the result images, initial calibration yields results that fit into the expected range of the values measured before. The chip and its cuboid shape are accurately reconstructed. The height, which is specified at around 6 mm according to the data-sheet is in the same range as the height computed by the presented method. When looking at Figure 3.1(c), it becomes evident that the calibration needs to be optimized as currently single outliers in the list of corresponding points result in a displacement of the estimated LED position, which directly influences height estimation. Another point for improvement is the shadow edge detection, as single artifacts worsen the measurement results. This cannot alone be achieved by changing the edge detection algorithms or further post-processing but needs to be incorporated into a model approach which uses sanity checks to remove falsely detected contours. As shown in Figure 3.1 on flat objects, that are known before hand, these calibration errors can be corrected after the reconstruction by averaging the height values. But for rough surfaces, this compensation approach will lower the reproduction granularity of the surface and therefore the height resolution will be further reduced. Hence it is suggested to reduce possible errors in each image processing step. When comparing the given results with the microscope's measurement one can see, that the height dimensions are in a similar range but still way off when micrometer accuracy is required. A really big advantage of the donated setup is the large lateral range $1000 \times 1000\ \mu\mathrm{m}^2$ that can be measured without stitching partial results together.

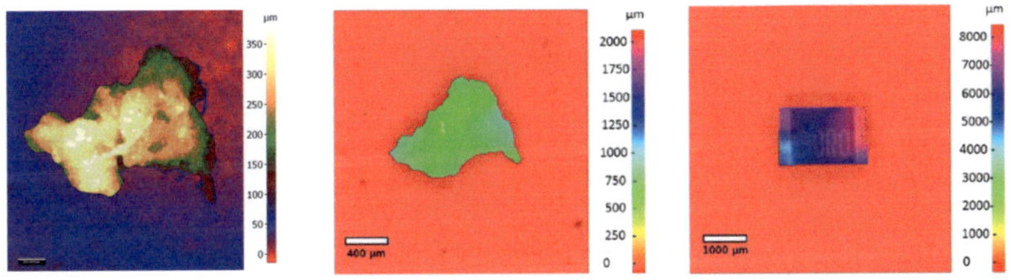

(a) (b) (c)

Figure 3.1: Alicona's InfiniteFocus reconstruction with clear surface details (a) and reconstructions estimated with the methods presented in this report (b) and(c).

4 Conclusion and discussion

There are two critical parts in this setup. The first part is for sure the initial calibration of the experimental setup, which will be examined in future research. The other critical part is the estimation of the shadow boundaries, because these directly influence the height estimation. In the presented approach every pixel is used with the same weight, meaning every pixel has the same impact in the algorithm to estimate the height values. As seen in Figure 4.1 the algorithm is very sensitive to noise. Every pixel, that is segmented from the background is directly added into the boundary list B_i and therefore used for computing the height-value. As of now there is no regularization that could work around wrongly detected pixels or noise. Figure 4.1(c) especially shows that noise will highly influence the measurement. As the noise has a large impact on the error, this issue violates the conditions of a well-posed problem, according to [Rie03] the given problem is ill-posed out of that reason. Future methods therefore need to propose a way for regularization. This could be by defining proximity rules for boundary pixel within a neighborhood. Fixating the area around a particle out of given geometric preconditions and the already known light position $\boldsymbol{L_i}$ is also suggested.

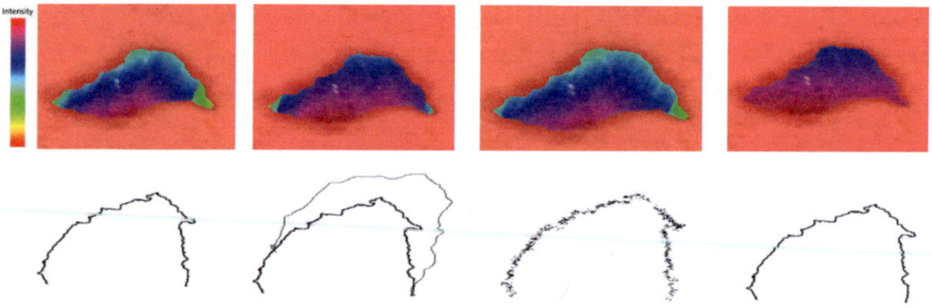

(a) (b) (c) (d)

Figure 4.1: From left to right the original contour (a) produced by $\boldsymbol{L_6}$ was modified by extending the original contour (b), adding noise around the contour (c) and by adding noise onto the complete image (d). All images are colored with the same color scale. All images use the same color-map and are directly comparable.

Besides the issues concerning robustness, the approach shown in section 2 is already producing results. It was implemented as a software and hardware prototype with the goal to realize a cost-efficient sensor for estimating height and volume information of dirt particles. As demonstrated in section 3, it is possible to estimate this information with a quite simple setup. In the future, these results need to be further compared and benchmarked in detail against ground-truth measurements to determine the accuracy and robustness of this approach. On the qualitative side the introduced model should also be extended by surface properties like roughness or material characteristics to improve the height estimation. The artifacts introduced by assuming a linear relation between shadow contour candidate, the point light position and the resulting height could be post-processed by introducing these surface characteristics.

Estimating height information while maintaining high-throughput measurements in the context of an industrial in-line QA process is still a critical task today. Hence a huge demand for measurement systems, that can ensure persistence in industrial environments while also keeping service costs low exists. The solution shown in this paper yields great potential for those kind of systems in the near future.

Bibliography

[BPLF12] Jürgen Beyerer, Fernando Puente León, and Christian Frese. *Automatische Sichtprüfung: Grundlagen, Methoden und Praxis der Bildgewinnung und Bildauswertung*. Springer Vieweg, 2012.

[Bra00] G. Bradski. *Dr. Dobb's Journal of Software Tools*, 2000.

[dA14] Verband der Automobilindustrie. *VDA Band 19 Püfung der Technischen Sauberkeit – Partikelverunreinigung funktionsrelevanter Automobilteile*, 2014.

[FKB14] Peter Frühberger, Edmund Klaus, and Jürgen Beyerer. Microscopic analysis using gaze-based interaction. volume 154 of *Springer Proceedings in Physics*, 2014.

[FSB15] Peter Frühberger, Thomas Stephan, and Jürgen Beyerer. Integrating microscopic analysis into existing quality assurance processes. volume 164 of *Springer Proceedings in Physics*, 2015.

[FSB16] Peter Frühberger, Thomas Stephan, and Jürgen Beyerer. Estimating 3d-volume of dirt particles using depth from shadow. volume 174 of *Springer Proceedings in Physics*, 2016. forthcoming.

[GW08] Rafael C. Gonzalez and Richard E. Woods. *Digital Image Processing*. Pearson International Edition, 3 edition, 2008.

[Rie03] Andreas Rieder. *Keine Probleme mit Inversen Problemen : eine Einführung in ihre stabile Lösung*. Vieweg, Wiesbaden, 1. aufl. edition, 2003.

Systematic Evaluation of Moving Object Detection Methods for Wide Area Motion Imagery

Lars Sommer

Vision and Fusion Laboratory
Institute for Anthropomatics
Karlsruhe Institute of Technology (KIT), Germany
lars.sommer@kit.edu

Technical Report IES-2015-12

Abstract: Wide area motion imagery (WAMI) facilitates the surveillance of several tens of square kilometers while using only one airborne sensor platform. Typical applications such as automatic behavior recognition, scene understanding, or traffic monitoring depend on precise multiple object tracking. Therefore, moving object detection is generally used as initial step. However, reliable moving object detection for WAMI is challenging as imprecise image alignment, low object resolution and a large number of moving objects lead to split, merged, and missing detections. In the context of this report, a detailed overview of existing methods for moving object detection proposed for WAMI is given. Ten existing methods as well as a novel combination of short-term background subtraction and suppression of image alignment errors by pixel neighborhood consideration are systematically evaluated on the WPAFB 2009 dataset that contains more than 160,000 ground truth detections. Parameters that contribute most to the performance of each method, the influence of related pre-processing steps as well as the impact of varying traffic density and scenery on the performance are discussed.

1 Introduction

In recent years, wide area motion imagery (WAMI) has been attracting an increased amount of research attention as WAMI enables large area surveillance while using only one airborne sensor platform. The sensor is comprised of a matrix of multiple cameras. Images of neighboring cameras with partially overlapping field of view are stitched to form the image with large ground coverage.

The stitched images are typically collected at 1-2 Hz due to the large volume (up to 100 megapixels). As WAMI data like the publicly available WPAFB 2009 dataset [U.S09] cover several tens of square kilometers and can contain thousands of moving objects per frame, applications such as driver behavior analysis or traffic monitoring are facilitated at large scale. These applications generally depend on multiple object tracking and consequently on object detections that are used at different stages in the tracking algorithm such as track initialization or object-to-track association [BTX+14]. Object detections are obtained by object segmentation approaches based frame differencing or background subtraction.

However, moving object detection in WAMI is very challenging: The moving objects are typically in the order of 10x20 pixels due to the low spatial resolution. Thus, detection approaches based on appearance features and machine learning are unreliable in WAMI so far [PM14]. The object detection is further complicated by weak contrast between object and background, shadows and occlusions that can lead to missed detections. Although image alignment is applied for camera motion compensation, residual errors of the alignment process as well as parallax effects can result in false positive detections. Additional challenges are sudden changes in camera gain and seam artifacts due to image stitching. Seam artifacts are caused by radiometric changes across different sensors and can produce false positive detections as sweeping seams can cause bands of large difference in the difference image [KGS13]. All these challenges can affect the performance of moving object detection. Nevertheless, there exists no systematic evaluation of moving object detection in WAMI so far even though missed detections emerge the need for track linking or false positive detections can cause the initialization of false positive tracks.

In this report, several moving object detection methods that are presented in WAMI literature are summarized and extended by a novel combination of short-term background subtraction and suppression of image alignment. In total, eleven methods are systematically evaluated on four image regions of the WPAFB 2009 dataset that comprises 1,025 frames. The different image regions contain more than 160,000 ground truth detections and offering different challenges such as traffic density and varying scenery.

2 Object Detection Methods

Object classification methods that are applied on WAMI data can be distinguished into frame differencing and background subtraction. As frame differencing requires less frames, residual errors of the alignment process are reduced compared to background subtraction [SS13]. A drawback of frame differencing compared to background subtraction is the sensitivity to detect slow moving objects whose positions partially overlap in consecutive frames and consequently can lead to missed detections. Further approaches that are widely used in aerial videos such as methods based on optical flow vectors and appearance feature based methods are not applicable [APK14] or unreliable [PM14], respectively. Thus, only frame differencing and background subtraction approaches that are presented in WAMI literature are summarized and discussed in the following subsections.

2.1 Frame Differencing

Moving object detection methods based on frame differencing can be classified into two-frame and three-frame differencing. Two-frame differencing calculates the pixel-wise intensity difference between two consecutive frames by:

$$D(x,y) = |I_t(x,y) - \hat{I}_{t-1}(x,y)|,$$

where $D(x,y)$ is the intensity value difference at pixel (x,y) and I_t and $\hat{I}_{t-1}$ denote the intensity values of frame t and the aligned frame $t-1$. The difference image for three-frame differencing is given by the minimum of the differnece image between frame t and $t-1$ and the difference image between frame t and $t+1$:

$$D(x,y) = \min(|I_t(x,y) - \hat{I}_{t-1}(x,y)|, |I_t(x,y) - \hat{I}_{t+1}(x,y)|)$$

As two-frame differencing requires only two consecutive frames, the residual errors of the alignment process are minimal. However, each moving object produces two motion blobs in the difference image. One blob represents the object position in the current frame and an additional one represents its position in the previous frame. Saleemi and Shah [SS13] applied two-frame differencing on WAMI data and proposed to handle this so called *ghosting effect* by rejecting blobs with smaller mean gradient magnitude and intensity standard deviation in the current frame compared to the previous frame. Xiao et al. [XCSH10] applied instead three-frame differencing to avoid multiple blobs for each moving object. Additional residual errors caused by the alignment process can be suppressed by using the minimum differences of each pixel in small neighborhoods as proposed by Pollard and Antone [PA12]. Keck et al. [KGS13] extended three-frame differencing by applying a box filter to the difference image to reduce false positive detections caused by seam artifacts.

2.2 Background Subtraction

In general, moving object detection based on background subtraction is performed by calculating the difference image $D(x, y)$ between an image I_t and its corresponding background model I_{BG}:

$$D(x, y) = \min(|I_t(x, y) - I_{BG}(x, y)|)$$

A straightforward method to acquire a background model is to calculate the pixel-wise intensity median of consecutive frames. The number of frames used for background modeling applied on WAMI data range from 8 [LLB$^+$13] to 16 [PDM11] and is thus clearly higher than the number of frames required for frame differencing. Incorporating background gradient information can be used to suppress noise in the difference image caused by parallax effects or residual errors due to the alignment process. Reilly et al. [RIS10] proposed to subtract the background gradient magnitudes from the difference images whereas Liang et al. [LLB$^+$13] modified this approach by replacing the subtraction with an additional threshold operation. Pixels that corresponding background magnitude exceeds a given threshold are expected as noise and set to 0 in the difference image.

Calculating the pixel-wise intensity mean of consecutive frames is not considered as this approach requires four times the number of frames than median background modeling for comparable results [RIS10]. Kent et al. [KMP$^+$12] proposed an alternative mean background approach. Instead of calculating the pixel-wise intensity mean of consecutive frames, Kent et al. [KMP$^+$12] proposed to calculate the running mean and the standard deviation with a recursive filter. Pixels considered as moving are detected by comparing the difference between the intensity value I_t and the local mean μ to a local threshold which is given by the standard deviation multiplied with a set scaling factor.

More sophisticated approaches such as Gaussian mixture models are inapplicable for object detection in WAMI due to the high number of required frames [RIS10] as well as the sensitivity to illumination changes [SS13], parallax and registration drift [PA12]. Pollard and Antone [PA12] replaced the traditional GMM with an Interval Gaussian Mixture Model (IGMM). Each pixel is described as an interval limited by a minimum value μ_{min} and maximum value μ_{max}, instead of modeling each pixel as a mixture of Gaussians. The interval boundaries for each pixel are continuously updated by incorporating the minimum and maximum intensity values in a small neighborhood around the pixel in the current frame. Pixels that deviate more than a single global standard deviation value σ from this interval are considered as pixels belonging to a moving object.

A static background model based on an inpainting algorithm is proposed by Aeschliman et al. [APK14] Therefore, pixels assigned as objects by an initial difference image between the current and the previous image as well as pixels that correspond to objects in the previous frame are replaced based on directional and smoothness constraints to complete the background model.

2.3 Proposed Method

The combination of median background modeling and neighborhood consideration is expected to be a powerful approach that has not been reported yet. Preliminary experiments indicated good recall values in case of median background subtraction even for sequences with slow moving objects whose positions partially overlap between consecutive frames. However, median background modeling causes a high number of false positive detections due to parallax effects and the image alignment process. Neighborhood consideration seems to be an appropriate alternative for incorporating background gradient information to suppress false positive detections as noise caused by parallax effects as well as image alignment are in the order of a few pixels. Thus, the intensity value difference $D(x, y)$ between the current frame I_t and the corresponding median background model I_{BG} is given by the minimum difference between pixel (x, y) in the current frame and all pixels (x_i, y_j) in a given neighborhood N of the background model:

$$D(x, y) = \min_{i,j}(|I_t(x, y) - I_{BG}(x_i, y_j)|)$$

3 Experimental Results

In total, eleven object detection methods are considered for the evaluation. An overview of these methods is listed in Table 3.1. The performance of the selected methods is evaluated on four image regions of the WPAFB 2009 dataset [U.S09]. The image regions are selected with regard to the image regions evaluated by Basharat et al. [BTX$^+$14] and Keck et al. [KGS13]. The WPAFB 2009 dataset comprises 1,025 frames with annotated GT. In the context of this report, stopping and parked objects are removed from the GT in order to determine the correct number of missing detections. The four image regions shown in Fig. 3.1 consist of 2,278×2,278 pixels and represent different challenges such as traffic density and varying scenery. The performance of each method is evaluated by means of

$$precision = \frac{TP}{FP + TP}$$

and

$$recall = \frac{TP}{TP + FN},$$

where TP, FP and FN are the number of true positive, false positive and false negative detections. In order to be consistent with the literature, the centroid of each blob is considered as a detection. Thus, each detection is represented by a point. Detections with annotated GT within a radius of 20 pixels are defined as TP otherwise as FP. GT objects without associated detection are defined as FN. The distance is set to 20 pixel, since GT annotations can differ from the center of the object. Furthermore, the blob centroid is often shifted from the annotated GT position due to appendant shadows.

Source	Object Detection Method
Saleemi [SS13]	2-frame Differencing + Ghost Handling
Xiao [XCSH10]	3-frame Differencing
Keck [KGS13]	3-frame Differencing + Box Filter
Pollard [PA12]	3-frame Differencing + Neighborhood
Pollard [PA12]	Interval Gaussian Mixture Model
Shi [SLBH12]	Median Background
Reilly [RIS10]	Median Background + Gradient Magnitude Suppression
Liang [LLB+13]	Median Background + Gradient Magnitude Thresholding
Kent [KMP+12]	Mean Background + Local Thresholding
Aeschliman [APK14]	Inpaint
Proposed	Median Background + Neighborhood

Table 3.1: Evaluated methods for moving object detection.

Prior to moving object detection, the camera motion is compensated by image alignment. After image alignment global histogram matching (HM) [GW02] is used to adjust camera gain and illumination variation, followed by local Gaussian mean filtering (MF) [SKS14] to reduce seam artifacts. Fig. 3.2 shows the impact of histogram matching and Gaussian mean filtering exemplarily for two-frame differencing by means of difference images. Large intensity differences are markedly reduced by HM (Fig. 3.2(b)) compared to no HM (Fig. 3.2(a)). However, the left image region still exhibits large differences in intensity. The reason for these differences is intensity discontinuities in the images due to stitching. These so called seam artifacts are suppressed by additional MF as depicted in Fig. 3.2(c). The impact of HM and MF on the performance is illustrated in

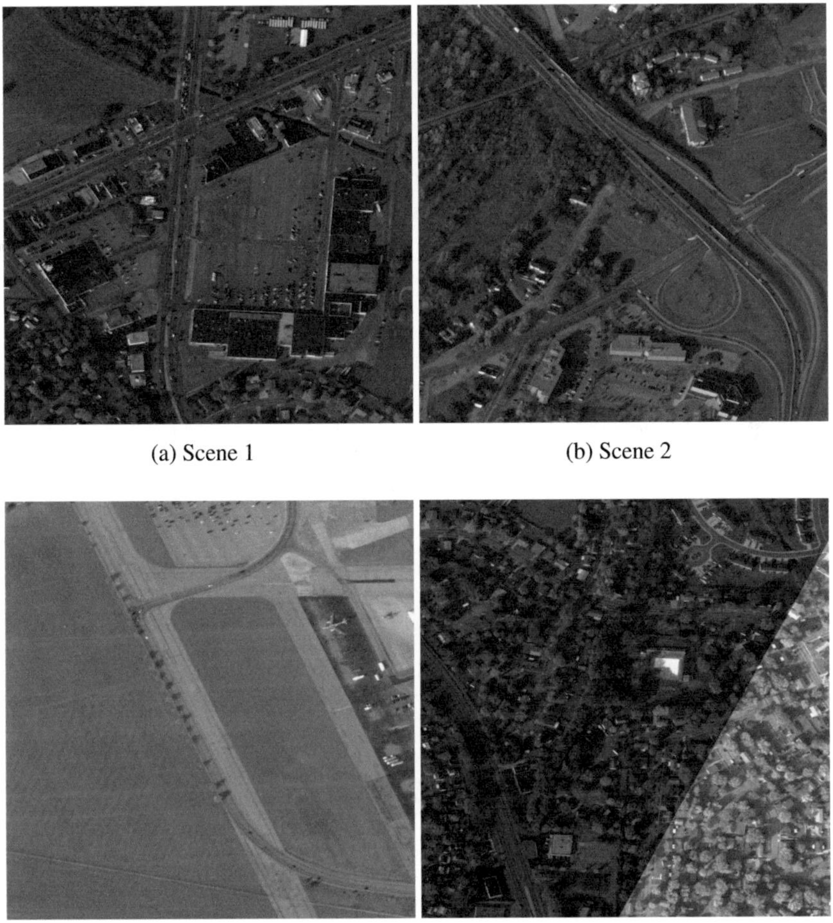

(a) Scene 1 (b) Scene 2

(c) Scene 3 (d) Scene 4

Figure 3.1: Image sections offering different challenges such as traffic density and varying scenery used for evaluation.

Fig. 3.3(a). As thresholding is used to distinguish pixels into objects and non-objects, it is expected that the threshold value has the highest impact on the performance. Thus, the shown precision-recall curves are generated by varying the

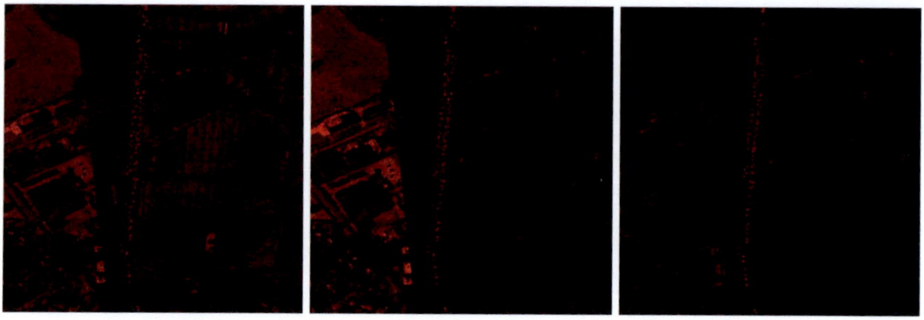

(a) no HM/MF (b) HM (c) HM+MF

Figure 3.2: Difference images for two-frame differencing without global histogram matching (HM) and local Gaussian mean filtering (MF) (a), with HM (b) and with HM and MF (c).

threshold value. The performance without HM and MF is considerably increased by applying HM whereas HM is outperformed by additional MF. Similar results are obtained for the other object detection methods as well for all scenes.

The performance of each object detection method is influenced by several parameters. The influence of relevant parameters is separately evaluated and optimized for each object detection method with regard to precision and recall. Thus, precision-recall curves are generated by varying the threshold value. In the following the parameters that contributed most to the performance are discussed. The corresponding precision-recall curves are given in Fig. 3.3(b)-3.3(f) exemplarily by means of scene 1.

In addition to the threshold value, all methods are affected by the minimum blob size. The minimum blob size is the minimal object size in pixels that is expected. Thus, detections with fewer pixels are associated as false detections and are rejected. The impact of the blob size on the performance of three-frame differencing is shown in Fig. 3.3(b). More false positives due to noise are rejected for larger minimum blob sizes. Consequently, the precision is increasing with increasing minimum blob sizes. In contrast, the recall is decreasing, since more small objects or partially detected objects are discarded.

The further parameters that are discussed are only relevant for particular methods. Methods based on median background modeling are affected by the number of frames used for modeling the median background. The precision-recall curve for various number of frames is depicted in Fig. 3.3(c). The precision is increasing

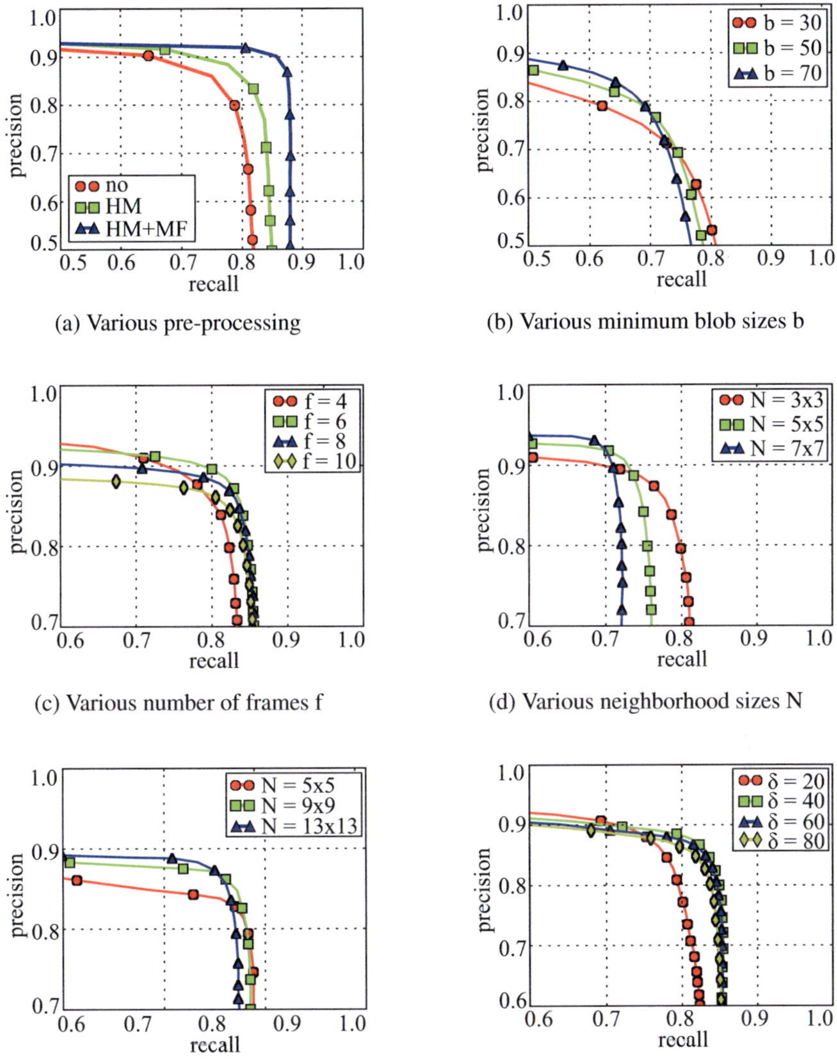

(a) Various pre-processing

(b) Various minimum blob sizes b

(c) Various number of frames f

(d) Various neighborhood sizes N

(e) Various neighborhood sizes N

(f) Various gradient thresholds δ

Figure 3.3: Variation of pre-processing steps (a) and optimization of parameters that contributed most to the object detection performance: (b) minimal blob size (in pixels), (c) number of frames used for median background modeling, (d)-(e) neighborhood size (in pixels) in case of 3-frame differencing and median background subtraction and (f) gradient magnitude threshold value δ in case of median background subtraction.

with fewer frames as the number of false positive detections caused by parallax effects or image alignment is reduced. The recall is almost the same for 6 to 10 frames. However, even less frames result in more missed detections. Reason for this is an inadequate estimated background especially in areas with dense traffic or intersections.

False positive detections caused by parallax effects or image alignment can be suppressed by neighborhood consideration. The impact of the applied neighborhood size on the performance of three-frame differencing and median background subtraction is shown in Fig. 3.3(d) and Fig. 3.3(e), respectively. More false positive detections are suppressed with increasing neighborhood sizes. However, the recall is decreasing with increasing neighborhood sizes as more small objects or partially detected objects are suppressed as well. Practical sizes are in the range of 3×3 to 5×5 pixels in case of three-frame differencing and slightly larger in case of median background subtraction as more errors are accumulated due to the number of used frames.

Background gradient information can be used to suppress false positive detections caused by parallax effects or image alignment as well. The impact of the gradient magnitude threshold δ on the performance of median background subtraction is illustrated in Fig. 3.3(f). As described in Section 2.2 gradient magnitudes above this threshold are expected to be caused by parallax and alignment errors and set to 0. The precision increases with lower threshold values as more errors are suppressed. In contrast, the recall is almost constant for threshold values between 40 and 80, but decreases considerably for lower threshold values as more objects are suppressed.

Fig. 3.4 shows the precision-recall curves of all methods for Scene 1-4. The parameters optimized for Scene 1 are adjusted for all Scenes. Median background subtraction without suppression of errors due to parallax effects or image alignment exhibits the worst performance of all methods for Scene 1,2,4. In contrast, the best performances are achieved for methods based on background subtraction that suppress these errors. Median background subtraction with neighborhood consideration outperforms both background gradient information based methods. Three-frame differencing with neighborhood consideration exhibits worse performance for Scene 1-3, whereas the performance is slightly better for Scene 4. The reason for the better performance is that Scene 4 showing a residential area densely covered with buildings and tree is more error prone to image alignment and parallax effects that are accumulated by the number of used frames. The weaker recall for Scene 1 indicates instead that median background models are more effective to detect slow moving objects especially in dense traffic. The other frame differencing methods show markedly worse performance compared

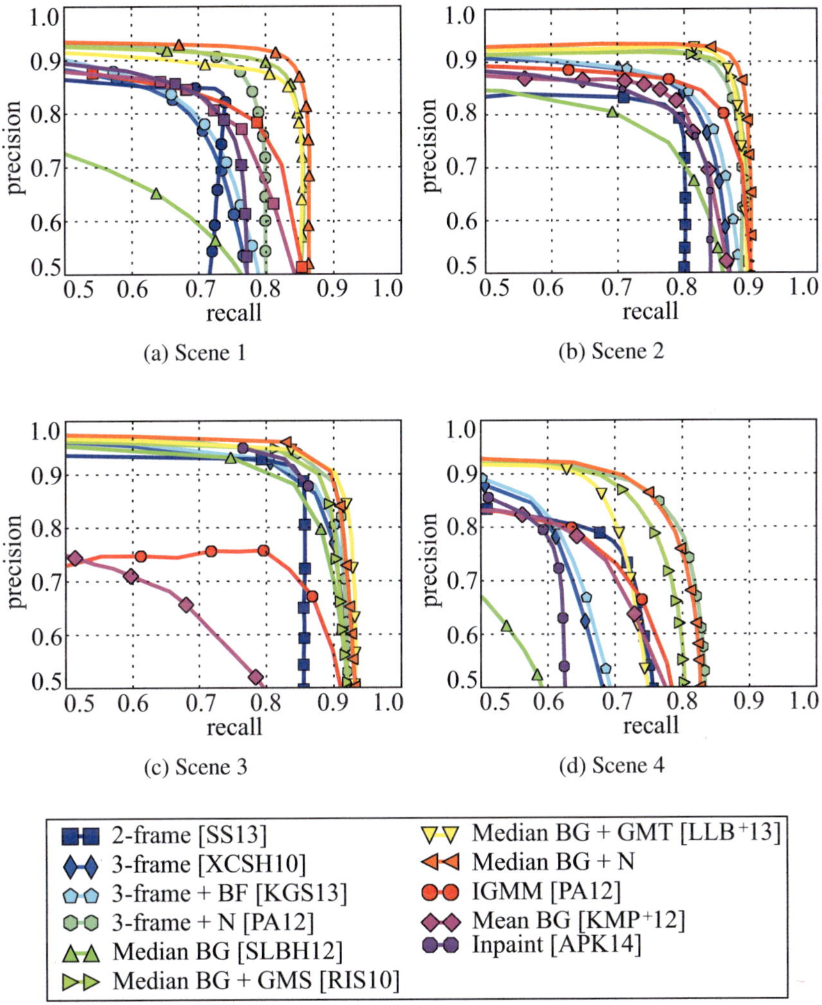

Figure 3.4: Precision-recall curves of all object detection methods for all four image regions.

to Three-frame differencing with neighborhood consideration. The impact of the locally applied box filter to suppress seam artifacts is marginal since these artifacts are partially suppressed during the pre-processing. The performance of the further background subtraction based methods is comparable to the frame differencing methods without neighborhood consideration except for Scene 3. The precision of IGMM for Scene 3 that is expected to be less challenging is considerably worse. The adaptive interval model and the fixed standard deviation used to segment pixels in object and non-object is not able to compensate for severe illumination changes and consequently results in a large number of false positive detections. The same difficulty is observed for the running mean approach which shows even poorer performance for this Scene.

4 Conclusion

In the context of this report, eleven object detection methods were evaluated on four different challenging image regions of the WPAFB 2009 dataset. For this purpose, the impact of pre-processing steps as well as parameters contributing most to the performance was discussed. The performance can be considerably increased by applying histogram matching and local Gaussian mean filtering to adjust camera gain and illumination variation and to suppress seam artifacts. The strong impact of various parameters on the object detection performance exhibits that the adjustment of these parameters is not neglible with regard to the following applications. The best performance overall is achieved by median background subtraction with neighborhood consideration that slightly outperforms other approaches for the suppression of errors caused by imprecise image alignment and parallax effects. The fact that other methods exhibit considerably worse performance indicates the importance of the suppression of these kinds of errors. Nevertheless, the impact of optimized moving object detection on existing multiple object tracking algorithms itself has to be analyzed.

Bibliography

[APK14] Chad Aeschliman, Johnny Park, and Avinash C. Kak. Tracking Vehicles Through Shadows and Occlusions in Wide-Area Aerial Video. *IEEE Transactions on Aerospace and Electronic Systems*, 50(1):429–444, 2014.

[BTX+14] Arslan Basharat, Matt Turek, Yiliang Xu, Chuck Atkins, David Stoup, Keith Fieldhouse, Paul Tunison, and Anthony Hoogs. Real-time Multi-Target Tracking at 210 Megapixels second in Wide Area Motion Imagery. *WACV*, pages 839–846, 2014.

[GW02] Rafael C. Gonzalez and Richard E. Woods. *Digital Image Processing*, pages 94–102. Prentice Hall, 2nd edition, 2002.

[KGS13] Mark Keck, Luis Galup, and Chris Stauffer. Real-time Tracking of Low-resolution Vehicles for Wide-Area Persistent Surveillance. In *WACV*, 2013.

[KMP+12] Phil Kent, Simon Maskell, Oliver Payne, Sean Richardson, and Larry Scarff. Robust Background Subtraction for Automated Detection and Tracking of Targets in Wide Area Motion Imagery. *Proc. SPIE*, 8546, 2012.

[LLB+13] Pengpeng Liang, Haibin Ling, Erik Blasch, Guna Seetharaman, Dan Shen, and Genshe Chen. Vehicle Detection in Wide Area Aerial Surveillance using Temporal Context. In *FUSION*, 2013.

[PA12] Thomas Pollard and Matthew Antone. Detecting and Tracking All Moving Objects in Wide-Area Aerial Video. In *CVPRW*, 2012.

[PDM11] Jan Prokaj, Mark Duchaineau, and Gerard Medioni. Inferring Tracklets for Multi-Object Tracking. In *CVPRW*, 2011.

[PM14] Jan Prokaj and Gerard Medioni. Persistent Tracking for Wide Area Aerial Surveillance. In *CVPR*, 2014.

[RIS10] Vladimir Reilly, Haroon Idrees, and Mubarak Shah. Detection and Tracking of Large Number of Targets in Wide Area Surveillance. In *ECCV*, 2010.

[SKS14] Günter Saur, Wolfgang Krüger, and Arne Schumann. Extended image differencing for change detection in UAV video mosaics. In *Proceedings of SPIE Vol. 9026*, 2014.

[SLBH12] Xinchu Shi, Haibin Ling, Erik Blasch, and Weiming Hu. Context-Driven Moving Vehicle Detection in Wide Area Motion Imagery. In *ICPR*, 2012.

[SS13] Imram Saleemi and Mubarak Shah. Multiframe Many-Many Point Correspondence for Vehicle Tracking in High Density Wide Area Aerial Videos. *IJCV*, 104(2):198–219, 2013.

[U.S09] U.S. Air Force Research Lab. SDMS: WPAFB 2009 Dataset. `https://www.sdms.afrl.af.mil/index.php?collection=wpafb2009`, 2009.

[XCSH10] Jiangjian Xiao, Hui Cheng, Harpreet Sawhney, and Feng Han. Vehicle Detection and Tracking in Wide Field-of-View Aerial Video. In *CVPR*, 2010.

Specular flow and Weingarten map

Alexey Pak

Vision and Fusion Laboratory
Institute for Anthropomatics
Karlsruhe Institute of Technology (KIT), Germany
apak@ies.uni-karlsruhe.de

Technical Report IES-2015-13

Abstract: If a moving camera observes a specular surface in which some environment is reflected, the pixel values per se do not directly characterise the surface. However, the associated optical flow, or specular flow (SF), as it is called in this situation, is an environment-agnostic observable that depends on the surface position, orientation, and curvature. The derivation of the SF in the limit of an infinitely remote environment has been published earlier by the authors, but in a relatively opaque coordinate-dependent form. In this report, we present a simpler and a more general derivation of the SF as a function of the surface structure, where the crucial part is played by the so-called Weingarten map. This result allows us to formulate the conditions when the SF diverges, and to derive a simple formula to relate the Gaussian curvature of the surface to the SF.

1 Introduction

The shape-from-specular flow (SFSF) approach has been suggested [RB06] as a convenient tool to estimate the 3D shape of moving reflecting objects while abstracting away from the details of the environment. One first estimates the optical flow (OF) field – the apparent displacements of prominent image elements between the subsequent video frames – and uses it to reconstruct the shape. If the camera observes a curved mirror, the motion field may exhibit smooth distortions, infinities, discontinuities etc., which may warrant the adaptation of the common OF algorithms. Such OF is commonly referred to as specular flow (SF) [AZBS11, CnVA$^+$09].

The first SFSF methods were able to estimate the parameters of simple known shapes [RB06]. Later, the problem was theoretically re-formulated in terms of global variational reconstruction [LBRB08]. More recently, Adato et al [AVBSZ07, AVZBS10, CnVA+09, VZGBS11] provided a practical general solution for a special setup where a telecentric camera is fixed with respect to the object and the infinitely remote textured environment undergoes a global rigid rotation. The flow field is obtained from the camera images with the common OF algorithms, and the resulting system of coupled linear partial differential equations is discretized and solved with standard tools. The improvements introduced in that series of papers lead to significant relaxation of the original requirements to the system calibration and the needed data, and reduced the problem to a system of linear partial differential equations (PDEs) [CnVA+09].

While very elegant, such an approach is not yet suitable for the common industrial settings. A more realistic setup would use e.g. a pinhole camera, moving along some trajectory with respect to the object that reflects a distant static environment. In this formulation, the problem has an additional dimensional parameter that is missing in the orthographic model – the distance between the camera and the object. The motion of isolated specularities relative to the fixed surface features in this case has been studied in [BB91], but no attempt has been made to recover the arbitrary surface shapes from the observed data. More recently, [Pak14a] introduced the paraxial formalism for the SF in perspective projection but did not present the final results.

In what follows we reproduce the derivation of the main results of [Pak14a] with the help of an alternative approach developed in [BB91]. We further analyze the structure of the resulting SF equations and in particular outline the relation between the Gaussian curvature of the surface and the observed specular flow.

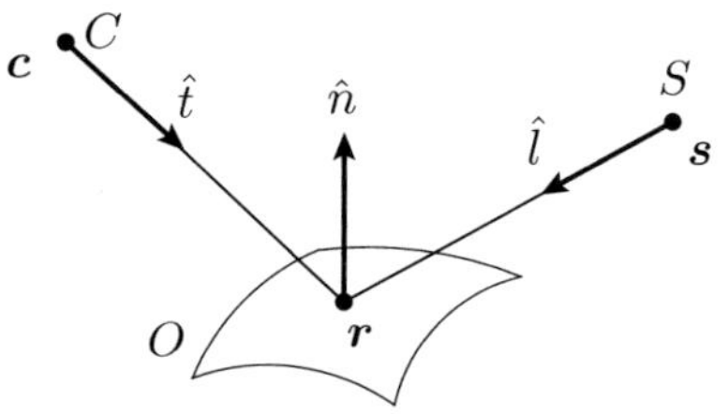

Figure 2.1: Geometry of a camera's view ray after a single specular reflection.

2 Notation

Let us assume an observation setup shown in Fig. 2.1. A camera C with the projection center located at point $\boldsymbol{c}$ observes a reflection of a light source S located at $\boldsymbol{s}$. A light ray originates at S and follows the (unit) direction $\hat{l}$ until it hits the specular object O at some surface point $\boldsymbol{r}$, and then reflects towards the camera. The unit direction from the camera to the reflection point is $\hat{t}$, and the normalized surface normal vector at the reflection point is $\hat{n}$. The distances from the camera and the source to the reflection point are λ and μ, respectively, i.e.

$$\boldsymbol{r} = \boldsymbol{c} + \lambda\,\hat{t} = \boldsymbol{s} + \mu\,\hat{l}. \tag{2.1}$$

In what follows, we will heavily use a linear operator $\pi[\hat{d}]$ that projects an arbitrary vector $\boldsymbol{x}$ on the subspace orthogonal to $\hat{d}$ (some unit vector such as $\hat{n}$, $\hat{t}$, or $\hat{l}$):

$$\pi[\hat{d}] \cdot \boldsymbol{x} \equiv \boldsymbol{x}_{\perp\hat{d}} = \boldsymbol{x} - \hat{d}\,(\boldsymbol{x}\cdot\hat{d}), \quad \text{or} \quad \left(\pi[\hat{d}]\right)_{ij} = \delta_{ij} - d_i d_j, \tag{2.2}$$

where δ_{ij} is the Kronecker symbol and d_i, d_j are the components of $\hat{d}$. For the product of two projectors, we reserve the special notation $\Pi = \pi[\hat{n}]\cdot\pi[\hat{t}]/\left(\hat{n}\cdot\hat{t}\right)$. We will also need a projector $\mathcal{P}$ whose action on a vector $\boldsymbol{x}$ is as follows:

$$\mathcal{P}\cdot\boldsymbol{x} = \frac{\hat{n}\times\left(\boldsymbol{x}\times\hat{t}\right)}{\hat{n}\cdot\hat{t}}, \quad \text{or} \quad (\mathcal{P})_{ij} = \delta_{ij} - \frac{t_i\,n_j}{\hat{n}\cdot\hat{t}}.$$

The latter expression may be obtained by contracting antisymmetric tensors[1] in the more explicit form $(\mathcal{P})_{ij} = \epsilon_{ikl}\,n_k\,\epsilon_{ljm}\,t_m/\left(\hat{n}\cdot\hat{t}\right)$. From the above definitions and the matrix forms of the projectors, one easily finds their trivial properties:

$$\pi[\hat{d}]\cdot\boldsymbol{x} = \boldsymbol{0} \text{ for } \boldsymbol{x} \parallel \hat{d}, \;\; \pi[\hat{d}]\cdot\boldsymbol{x} = \boldsymbol{x} \text{ for } \boldsymbol{x}\perp\hat{d}, \tag{2.3}$$
$$\mathcal{P}\cdot\boldsymbol{x} = \boldsymbol{0} \text{ for } \boldsymbol{x}\parallel\hat{t}, \;\; \mathcal{P}\cdot\boldsymbol{x} = \boldsymbol{x} \text{ for } \boldsymbol{x}\perp\hat{n}, \;\; \mathcal{P}\cdot\pi[\hat{t}] = \mathcal{P}, \text{ and } \Pi\cdot\mathcal{P} = \Pi.$$

Since the SF is related to motion, we use the "dotted"notation for time derivatives. For example, the camera's velocity is $\dot{\boldsymbol{c}} \equiv \partial\boldsymbol{c}/\partial t$. In a scene of Fig. 2.1, in general, if the camera moves, only the source location remains constant, i.e. $\dot{\boldsymbol{s}} \equiv \boldsymbol{0}$.

[1] A fully antisymmetric tensor, or a Levi-Civita symbol, is defined here as follows: $\epsilon_{123} = 1$, and $\epsilon_{ijk} = -\epsilon_{jik} = -\epsilon_{ikj}$. It is commonly used to define vector products: $(\boldsymbol{a}\times\boldsymbol{b})_i = \epsilon_{ijk}a_j b_k$.

Finally, we introduce the Weingarten map W that connects the variation of a point $\boldsymbol{r}$ on a surface and the respective change in the normal vector $\hat{n}$. In particular,

$$\dot{\hat{n}} = W \cdot \dot{\boldsymbol{r}}. \tag{2.4}$$

The coordinate representation of W is frame-dependent, but its eigenvalues and eigenvectors are the intrinsic invariant properties of the surface at the point $\boldsymbol{r}$.

3 Specular flow for a moving pinhole camera

With the introduced notation, we are now in the position to derive the specular flow perceived by the moving camera (the object O and the source S remain static) in terms of the camera motion $\dot{\boldsymbol{c}}$ and the local surface parameters at point $\boldsymbol{r}$. Our guideline will be to prevent the proliferation of the source parameters to the result.

According to Fig. 2.1, the directions $\hat{t}$, $\hat{s}$, and $\hat{n}$ satisfy the reflection law, i.e.

$$\hat{t} + \hat{l} = \nu\, \hat{n} \tag{3.1}$$

for some ν. Let us differentiate Eq. (3.1) with respect to time and apply $\pi[\hat{n}]$:

$$\pi[\hat{n}] \cdot \left(\dot{\hat{t}} + \dot{\hat{l}}\right) = \pi[\hat{n}] \cdot \left(\dot{\nu}\, \hat{n} + \nu\, \dot{\hat{n}}\right) = \nu\, \dot{\hat{n}}. \tag{3.2}$$

The latter equality holds since $\|\hat{n}\| = 1$, thus $\dot{\hat{n}} \cdot \hat{n} = 0$ and $\pi[\hat{n}] \cdot \dot{\hat{n}} = \dot{\hat{n}}$. Next, let us multiply Eq. (3.1) with $\hat{n}$ and use $\hat{n} \cdot \hat{t} = \hat{n} \cdot \hat{l}$:

$$\nu = \hat{n} \cdot \left(\hat{t} + \hat{l}\right) = 2\hat{n} \cdot \hat{t}. \tag{3.3}$$

Substituting ν from Eq. (3.3) into Eq. (3.2), we arrive at

$$\dot{\hat{n}} = \pi[\hat{n}] \cdot \left(\dot{\hat{t}} + \dot{\hat{l}}\right) / \left(2\hat{n} \cdot \hat{t}\right). \tag{3.4}$$

Next, let us differentiate the first equality in Eq. (2.1) and project it using $\pi[\hat{t}]$:

$$\pi[\hat{t}] \cdot \dot{\boldsymbol{r}} = \pi[\hat{t}] \cdot \left(\dot{\boldsymbol{c}} + \dot{\lambda}\, \hat{t} + \lambda\, \dot{\hat{t}}\right) = \pi[\hat{t}] \cdot \dot{\boldsymbol{c}} + \lambda\, \dot{\hat{t}}, \text{ or}$$

$$\dot{\hat{t}} = \lambda^{-1} \pi[\hat{t}] \cdot \left(\dot{\boldsymbol{r}} - \dot{\boldsymbol{c}}\right). \tag{3.5}$$

Again, we exploit that $\dot{\hat{t}} \cdot \hat{t} = 0$ and $\pi[\hat{t}] \cdot \dot{\hat{t}} = \dot{\hat{t}}$. By analogy, we may differentiate the second equality of Eq. (2.1), project it with $\pi[\hat{l}]$, and use $\dot{\boldsymbol{s}} \equiv \boldsymbol{0}$ to find

$$\dot{\hat{l}} = \mu^{-1} \pi[\hat{l}] \cdot \dot{\boldsymbol{r}}. \tag{3.6}$$

Now we may substitute Eqs. (3.5) and (3.6) into Eq. (3.4):

$$\dot{\hat{n}} = \pi[\hat{n}] \cdot \left[\lambda^{-1}\pi[\hat{t}] \cdot (\dot{\boldsymbol{r}} - \dot{\boldsymbol{c}}) + \mu^{-1}\pi[\hat{l}] \cdot \dot{\boldsymbol{r}}\right] / \left(2\hat{n} \cdot \hat{t}\right). \tag{3.7}$$

This expression involves the operator products $\pi[\hat{n}] \cdot \pi[\hat{t}]$ and $\pi[\hat{n}] \cdot \pi[\hat{l}]$. In order to eliminate the source-dependent operator $\pi[\hat{l}]$, we must prove that

$$\pi[\hat{n}] \cdot \pi[\hat{l}] \cdot \dot{\boldsymbol{r}} = \pi[\hat{n}] \cdot \pi[\hat{t}] \cdot \dot{\boldsymbol{r}}. \tag{3.8}$$

Indeed, since $\dot{\boldsymbol{r}}$ is tangential, and $\hat{n}$ is orthogonal to the mirror surface, then $\dot{\boldsymbol{r}} \cdot \hat{n} = 0$. Further, the reflection law Eq. (3.1) implies that $\hat{t} = \boldsymbol{t}_{\|\hat{n}} + \boldsymbol{t}_{\perp\hat{n}}$ and $\hat{l} = \boldsymbol{t}_{\|\hat{n}} - \boldsymbol{t}_{\perp\hat{n}}$, where $\hat{n} \cdot \boldsymbol{t}_{\perp\hat{n}} = 0$ and $\boldsymbol{t}_{\|\hat{n}} = (\nu/2)\,\hat{n}$. Combined, this leads to the equality

$$\hat{t} \cdot \dot{\boldsymbol{r}} = \boldsymbol{t}_{\perp\hat{n}} \cdot \dot{\boldsymbol{r}} = -\hat{l} \cdot \dot{\boldsymbol{r}}. \tag{3.9}$$

Using Eq. (2.2) and (3.9), we than establish that

$$\pi[\hat{n}] \cdot \pi[\hat{t}] \cdot \dot{\boldsymbol{r}} = \pi[\hat{n}] \cdot \left[\dot{\boldsymbol{r}} - \hat{t}\left(\hat{t} \cdot \dot{\boldsymbol{r}}\right)\right] = \dot{\boldsymbol{r}} - \boldsymbol{t}_{\perp\hat{n}}\left(\hat{t} \cdot \dot{\boldsymbol{r}}\right), \text{ and}$$
$$\pi[\hat{n}] \cdot \pi[\hat{l}] \cdot \dot{\boldsymbol{r}} = \pi[\hat{n}] \cdot \left[\dot{\boldsymbol{r}} - \hat{l}\left(\hat{l} \cdot \dot{\boldsymbol{r}}\right)\right] = \dot{\boldsymbol{r}} + \boldsymbol{t}_{\perp\hat{n}}\left(\hat{l} \cdot \dot{\boldsymbol{r}}\right) = \dot{\boldsymbol{r}} - \boldsymbol{t}_{\perp\hat{n}}\left(\hat{t} \cdot \dot{\boldsymbol{r}}\right).$$

This proves Eq. (3.8) and allows us to transform Eq. (3.7) into

$$\dot{\hat{n}} = \pi[\hat{n}] \cdot \pi[\hat{t}] \cdot \left[\lambda^{-1}\left(\dot{\boldsymbol{r}} - \dot{\boldsymbol{c}}\right) + \mu^{-1}\dot{\boldsymbol{r}}\right] / \left(2\hat{n} \cdot \hat{t}\right). \tag{3.10}$$

Our primary quantity of interest is the SF, defined as $\boldsymbol{f} \equiv \dot{\hat{t}}$, i.e. it is the variation of the sight ray direction caused by the motion of the camera. From Eq. (3.5),

$$\lambda\,\boldsymbol{f} = \pi[\hat{t}] \cdot (\dot{\boldsymbol{r}} - \dot{\boldsymbol{c}}). \tag{3.11}$$

Applying $\mathcal{P}$ on Eq. (3.11), using Eq. (2.3) and the fact that $\dot{\boldsymbol{r}} \perp \hat{n}$, we find:

$$\lambda\mathcal{P} \cdot \boldsymbol{f} = \mathcal{P} \cdot \pi[\hat{t}] \cdot (\dot{\boldsymbol{r}} - \dot{\boldsymbol{c}}) = \dot{\boldsymbol{r}} - \mathcal{P} \cdot \dot{\boldsymbol{c}}, \quad \text{or} \quad \dot{\boldsymbol{r}} = \mathcal{P} \cdot (\lambda\boldsymbol{f} + \dot{\boldsymbol{c}}). \tag{3.12}$$

Now we may plug $\dot{\hat{n}}$ of Eq. (2.4) and $\dot{\boldsymbol{r}}$ of Eq. (3.12) into Eq. (3.10) and simplify:

$$\dot{\hat{n}} = W \cdot \dot{\boldsymbol{r}} = W \cdot \mathcal{P} \cdot (\lambda\boldsymbol{f} + \dot{\boldsymbol{c}}) = \frac{1}{2}\,\Pi \cdot \left[\kappa\,\mathcal{P} \cdot (\lambda\boldsymbol{f} + \dot{\boldsymbol{c}}) - \frac{\dot{\boldsymbol{c}}}{\lambda}\right], \text{ and}$$
$$\lambda^2\left[2W - \kappa\Pi\right] \cdot \mathcal{P} \cdot \boldsymbol{f} = \left[-2\lambda W \cdot \mathcal{P} + \lambda\kappa\Pi \cdot \mathcal{P} - \Pi\right] \cdot \dot{\boldsymbol{c}}.$$

(In the above formula, we introduce $\kappa = \lambda^{-1} + \mu^{-1}$). Using again the properties of the projectors Eq. (2.3), we arrive at the final invariant SF equation:

$$\lambda^2 \left[2W - \kappa\Pi\right] \cdot \mathcal{P} \cdot \boldsymbol{f} = \left[(\lambda\kappa - 1)\,\Pi - 2\lambda W \cdot \mathcal{P}\right] \cdot \dot{\boldsymbol{c}}. \tag{3.13}$$

In case the source S is located very far away from the mirror and the camera ($\mu \to \infty$), then $\kappa = \lambda^{-1}$, and we obtain an even simpler expression

$$\left[2\lambda W - \Pi\right] \cdot \mathcal{P} \cdot \boldsymbol{f} = -2W \cdot \mathcal{P} \cdot \dot{\boldsymbol{c}}.$$

4 Two-dimensional SF equation

First of all, we notice that Eq. (3.13) is linear in the SF and the camera velocity, as should be expected from the lowest-order approximation. Further, since both $\dot{\boldsymbol{c}}$ and $\boldsymbol{f}$ are multiplied with $\mathcal{P}$ or Π, their components parallel to $\hat{t}$ do not play any role, and Eq. (3.13) is equivalent to a system of two equations. We therefore cannot e.g. solve Eq. (3.13) for $\boldsymbol{f}$, since the matrix $[2W - \kappa\Pi] \cdot \mathcal{P}$ has no inverse.

In order to move further, let us assume some coordinate frame such that $\boldsymbol{c} = (0, 0, 0)^T$ and $\hat{t} = (0, 0, 1)^T$. The SF and the camera motion in this frame are $\boldsymbol{f} = (f_1, f_2, f_3)^T$ and $\dot{\boldsymbol{c}} = (\dot{c}_1, \dot{c}_2, \dot{c}_3)^T$. Since only the components of $\boldsymbol{f}$, $\dot{\boldsymbol{c}}$ orthogonal to $\hat{t}$ (i.e. the first and the second) matter, we may re-write Eq. (3.13) as follows:

$$\lambda^2 \left[2W_{(2)} - \kappa\Pi_{(2)}\right] \cdot \boldsymbol{f}_{(2)} = \left[(\lambda\kappa - 1)\,\Pi_{(2)} - 2\lambda W_{(2)}\right] \cdot \dot{\boldsymbol{c}}_{(2)}. \tag{4.1}$$

Here $\boldsymbol{f}_{(2)} = (f_1, f_2)^T$, $\dot{\boldsymbol{c}}_{(2)} = (\dot{c}_1, \dot{c}_2)^T$, and all operators with subscript (2) are 2×2 matrices obtained by dropping the last row and the last column from the 3×3 representation. In particular, $\mathcal{P}_{(2)}$ becomes a unit matrix and drops out, and $W_{(2)}$ is a matrix known as the second fundamental form of the surface.

Since the SF equation is two-dimensional, we may at any camera position record at most two independent SF vectors $\boldsymbol{f}_{(2)}^{(1)}$ and $\boldsymbol{f}_{(2)}^{(2)}$, corresponding to the two independent motion vectors $\dot{\boldsymbol{c}}_{(2)}^{(1)}$ and $\dot{\boldsymbol{c}}_{(2)}^{(2)}$. Having made two such observations, we combine them into the matrices $F = \left(\boldsymbol{f}_{(2)}^{(1)}, \boldsymbol{f}_{(2)}^{(2)}\right)$ and $\dot{C} = \left(\dot{\boldsymbol{c}}_{(2)}^{(1)}, \dot{\boldsymbol{c}}_{(2)}^{(2)}\right)$ so that

$$\lambda^2 \left[2W_{(2)} - \kappa\Pi_{(2)}\right] \cdot \tilde{F} = (\lambda\kappa - 1)\,\Pi_{(2)} - 2\lambda W_{(2)}, \tag{4.2}$$

where $\tilde{F} = F \cdot \left(\dot{C}\right)^{-1}$ is a normalized SF corresponding to the two orthogonal unit camera motions. Now the criterion for the existence of a finite SF is straightforward: if the matrix $\left[2W_{(2)} - \kappa\Pi_{(2)}\right]$ is singular, the SF diverges. This happens, when κ is an eigenvalue of the matrix $2W_{(2)} \cdot \Pi_{(2)}^{-1}$. Such condition is more complex than the identification of "parabolic points", commonly believed to cause infinite SF, and involves (via κ) the positions of the camera and the source.

In case $\mu \to \infty$ Eq. (4.2) simplifies to:

$$\left[2\lambda W_{(2)} - \Pi_{(2)}\right] \cdot \tilde{F} = -2W_{(2)}. \tag{4.3}$$

5 Gaussian curvature and the SF

Let us re-write Eq. (4.2) as

$$2\lambda W_{(2)} \cdot \left[\lambda\tilde{F} + I_{(2)}\right] = \Pi_{(2)} \cdot \left[(\lambda\kappa - 1)I_{(2)} + \lambda^2\kappa\tilde{F}\right], \tag{5.1}$$

where $I_{(2)}$ is a 2×2 unit matrix. If we introduce explicitly the components of the unit normal vector $\hat{n} = (n_1, n_2, n_3)^T$, the projector becomes

$$\Pi_{(2)} = \frac{1}{n_3}\begin{pmatrix} 1 - n_1^2 & -n_1 n_2 \\ -n_1 n_2 & 1 - n_2^2, \end{pmatrix},$$

which implies $\det \Pi_{(2)} = 1$. Taking the determinant of Eq. (5.1), we end up with

$$\det W_{(2)} = \det\left[(\lambda\kappa - 1)I_{(2)} + \lambda^2\kappa\tilde{F}\right] \det\left[2\lambda\left(\lambda\tilde{F} + I_{(2)}\right)\right]^{-1},$$

or, in the limit $\mu \to \infty$,

$$\det W_{(2)} = \det\left[\tilde{F}\right] \det\left[2\left(\lambda\tilde{F} + I_{(2)}\right)\right]^{-1}. \tag{5.2}$$

Eq. (5.2) is quite remarkable: $\det W_{(2)}$ is the Gaussian curvature, which is an intrinsic property of the surface at point $\boldsymbol{r}$, independent of how the surface is embedded in the 3D space. The right-hand side depends only on the measured SF matrix $\tilde{F}$ and the distance λ. Let us now consider three special cases:

- If the surface is nearly flat, the observed SF should be close to zero, and $\|\lambda\tilde{F}\| \ll 1$. The distance-dependent term then drops out, and we get

  $$\det W_{(2)} = \frac{1}{4}\det\tilde{F}.$$

  This equation suggests a direct method to measure small residual curvatures of nearly planar surfaces.

- If instead $\|\lambda\tilde{F}\| \gg 1$, which happens e.g. for a camera positioned near the focus point of a spherical mirror of radius 2λ (i.e. all camera sight rays are reflected in the same direction), the SF-dependence disappears, as expected:

$$\det W_{(2)} = \frac{1}{4\lambda^2}.$$

- If the surface is developable, i.e. it may be locally "unfolded" into a flat sheet without stretching (this happens when it is locally a cylinder), its Gaussian curvature is zero. According to Eq. 5.2, this implies that $\det \tilde{F} = 0$. The two recorded SF vectors then must be collinear, or, alternatively, there must exist a direction of the camera motion such that the respective SF vanishes. Intuitively, if the camera moves along the cylinder axis, then indeed the reflection of the infinitely remote environment must remain static on the sensor, and the SF is zero.

On a more general level, the derived relations between the SF and the curvature allow us to differentiate the SF-based reconstruction from the other optical shape measurement techniques as follows. The triangulation-based methods (as well as interferometry) are directly sensitive to the point position in space (or the zeroth-order derivative). In deflectometry, the primary measured quantity is the normal vector (the first-order surface derivatives). The SF, as shown above, is directly sensitive to the second order derivatives which enter the Weingarten map and the curvatures. Therefore, the error profiles and the dominant error sources of any SF-based methods will be different from the alternatives and may justify their use in some applications.

6 Explicit coordinate form

In order to obtain the explicit expressions for the Weingarten map and the normal vector, we need to assume some parametrization of the reflecting surface near $\boldsymbol{r}$ in terms of two intrinsic surface coordinates u and v. Given some function $\boldsymbol{r}(u, v)$,

$$W_{(2)} = \frac{1}{EG - F^2} \begin{pmatrix} eG - fF & fG - gF \\ fE - eF & gE - fF \end{pmatrix},$$

where $E = \boldsymbol{r}_u \cdot \boldsymbol{r}_u$, $F = \boldsymbol{r}_u \cdot \boldsymbol{r}_v$, $G = \boldsymbol{r}_v \cdot \boldsymbol{r}_v$, $e = \boldsymbol{r}_{uu} \cdot \hat{n}$, $f = \boldsymbol{r}_{uv} \cdot \hat{n}$, $g = \boldsymbol{r}_{vv} \cdot \hat{n}$, and the subscripts stand for the partial derivatives such as $\boldsymbol{r}_{uv} \equiv \partial_u \partial_v \boldsymbol{r}$.

One convenient parametrization identifies u and v with the sensor coordinates of a pinhole camera located at $\boldsymbol{c}$ such that its central direction coincides with $\hat{t}$, and the u- and v-axes are collinear with the global x- and y-axes, respectively. The surface geometry near $\boldsymbol{r}(0,0)$ is described by a two-dimensional depth map $s(u,v)$:

$$\boldsymbol{r}(u,v) = s(u,v)\,(u,v,1)^T, \text{where}$$
$$s(u,v) = s_0 + us_u + vs_v + \frac{u^2}{2}s_{uu} + \frac{v^2}{2}s_{vv} + uv\,s_{uv}.$$

This is precisely the parametrization suggested in [Pak14a]. If one expresses $W_{(2)}$ and the components of the normal vector $\hat{n} = (\boldsymbol{r}_v \times \boldsymbol{r}_u)/|\boldsymbol{r}_v \times \boldsymbol{r}_u|$ in terms of the shape parameters s_0, ..., s_{uv}, and substitutes them into Eq. (4.1) in the limit $\mu \to \infty$, one arrives at the explicit form of variables and the operators in Eq. (4.3):

$$\lambda = s_0,\;\; W_{(2)} = s^{-1}\left(s_0^2 + s_u^2 + s_v^2\right)^{-3/2} M, \text{ where}$$
$$M = s_0^2\begin{pmatrix} s_{uu} & s_{uv} \\ s_{uv} & s_{vv}\end{pmatrix} - 2s_0\begin{pmatrix} s_u^2 & s_u s_v \\ s_u s_v & s_v^2\end{pmatrix}$$
$$+\begin{pmatrix} s_v\left(s_v s_{uu} - s_u s_{uv}\right) & s_v\left(s_v s_{uv} - s_u s_{vv}\right) \\ -s_u\left(s_v s_{uu} - s_u s_{uv}\right) & -s_u\left(s_v s_{uv} - s_u s_{vv}\right)\end{pmatrix}, \text{ and}$$
$$\Pi_{(2)} = s^{-1}\left(s_0^2 + s_u^2 + s_v^2\right)^{-1/2}\begin{pmatrix} -s_0^2 - s_v^2 & s_u s_v \\ s_u s_v & -s_0^2 - s_u^2\end{pmatrix}.$$

Solving Eq. (4.1) with these operators for the components of $\boldsymbol{f}_{(2)}$ as a function of $\dot{\boldsymbol{c}}_{(2)}$, one exactly reproduces $\boldsymbol{f}(0,0)$ in Eq. (3.1) of that reference. Our present calculation is therefore equally powerful, but provides more insight into the structure of the SF equations.

7 Conclusion

In this report, we provided a detailed derivation of how the SF in a point depends on the observation parameters and the properties of the reflecting surface. Unlike previous results, the presented equations are explicitly invariant and compact, allowing a deeper insight into their structure. In particular, we formulated the simple condition for the SF to diverge, and highlighted the relation between the SF and the Gaussian curvature of the surface. The future work will be related to finding ways to recover the 3D shape of the surface based on the observed SF.

Bibliography

[AVBSZ07] Yair Adato, Yuriy Vasilyev, Ohad Ben-Shahar, and Todd Zickler. Toward a theory of shape from specular flow. Proc. ICCV, 2007.

[AVZBS10] Yair Adato, Yuriy Vasilyev, Todd Zickler, and Ohad Ben-Shahar. Shape from specular flow. *IEEE Trans. Pattern Anal. Mach. Intell.*, 32:2054 – 2070, 2010.

[AZBS11] Yair Adato, Todd Zickler, and Ohad Ben-Shahar. A polar representation of motion and implications for optical flow. Proc. CVPR, 2011.

[BB91] Andrew Blake and Heinrich Bülthoff. Shape from specularities: Computation and psychophysics. *Phil. Trans. R. Soc. Lond. B*, 331:237–252, 1991.

[CnVA+09] Guillermo D. Cañas, Yuriy Vasilyev, Yair Adato, Todd Zickler, Steven J. Gortler, and Ohad Ben-Shahar. A linear formulation of shape from specular flow. Proc. ICCV, pages 191–198, 2009.

[LBRB08] J. Lellmann, J. Balzer, A. Rieder, and J. Beyerer. Shape from specular reflection and optical flow. *Int J. Comput. Vis.*, 80:226–241, 2008.

[Pak14a] Alexey Pak. Local shape from specular flow. Proc. 2013 Joint Workshop of Fraunhofer IOSB and Institute for Anthropomatics, Vision and Fusion Laboratory, pages 53–59, 2014.

[RB06] Stefan Roth and Michael J. Black. Specular flow and the recovery of surface structure. Proc. CVPR, pages 1869–1876, 2006.

[VZGBS11] Yuriy Vasilyev, Todd Zickler, Steven Gortler, and Ohad Ben-Shahar. Shape from specular flow: Is one flow enough? Proc. CVPR, pages 2561–2568, 2011.

Karlsruher Schriftenreihe zur Anthropomatik
(ISSN 1863-6489)

Herausgeber: Prof. Dr.-Ing. Jürgen Beyerer

Die Bände sind unter www.ksp.kit.edu als PDF frei verfügbar
oder als Druckausgabe bestellbar.

Band 1 Jürgen Geisler
Leistung des Menschen am Bildschirmarbeitsplatz. 2006
ISBN 3-86644-070-7

Band 2 Elisabeth Peinsipp-Byma
Leistungserhöhung durch Assistenz in interaktiven Systemen zur Szenenanalyse. 2007
ISBN 978-3-86644-149-1

Band 3 Jürgen Geisler, Jürgen Beyerer (Hrsg.)
Mensch-Maschine-Systeme. 2010
ISBN 978-3-86644-457-7

Band 4 Jürgen Beyerer, Marco Huber (Hrsg.)
Proceedings of the 2009 Joint Workshop of Fraunhofer IOSB and Institute for Anthropomatics, Vision and Fusion Laboratory. 2010
ISBN 978-3-86644-469-0

Band 5 Thomas Usländer
Service-oriented design of environmental information systems. 2010
ISBN 978-3-86644-499-7

Band 6 Giulio Milighetti
Multisensorielle diskret-kontinuierliche Überwachung und Regelung humanoider Roboter. 2010
ISBN 978-3-86644-568-0

Band 7 Jürgen Beyerer, Marco Huber (Hrsg.)
Proceedings of the 2010 Joint Workshop of Fraunhofer IOSB and Institute for Anthropomatics, Vision and Fusion Laboratory. 2011
ISBN 978-3-86644-609-0

Band 8 Eduardo Monari
Dynamische Sensorselektion zur auftragsorientierten Objektverfolgung in Kameranetzwerken. 2011
ISBN 978-3-86644-729-5

Band 9 Thomas Bader
Multimodale Interaktion in Multi-Display-Umgebungen. 2011
ISBN 3-86644-760-8

Band 10 Christian Frese
Planung kooperativer Fahrmanöver für kognitive Automobile. 2012
ISBN 978-3-86644-798-1

Band 11 Jürgen Beyerer, Alexey Pak (Hrsg.)
Proceedings of the 2011 Joint Workshop of Fraunhofer IOSB and Institute for Anthropomatics, Vision and Fusion Laboratory. 2012
ISBN 978-3-86644-855-1

Band 12 Miriam Schleipen
Adaptivität und Interoperabilität von Manufacturing Execution Systemen (MES). 2013
ISBN 978-3-86644-955-8

Band 13 Jürgen Beyerer, Alexey Pak (Hrsg.)
Proceedings of the 2012 Joint Workshop of Fraunhofer IOSB and Institute for Anthropomatics, Vision and Fusion Laboratory. 2013
ISBN 978-3-86644-988-6

Band 14 Hauke-Hendrik Vagts
Privatheit und Datenschutz in der intelligenten Überwachung: Ein datenschutzgewährendes System, entworfen nach dem „Privacy by Design" Prinzip. 2013
ISBN 978-3-7315-0041-4

Band 15 Christian Kühnert
Data-driven Methods for Fault Localization in Process Technology. 2013
ISBN 978-3-7315-0098-8

Band 16 Alexander Bauer
Probabilistische Szenenmodelle für die Luftbildauswertung. 2014
ISBN 978-3-7315-0167-1

Band 17 Jürgen Beyerer, Alexey Pak (Hrsg.)
Proceedings of the 2013 Joint Workshop of Fraunhofer IOSB and Institute for Anthropomatics, Vision and Fusion Laboratory. 2014
ISBN 978-3-7315-0212-8

Band 18 Michael Teutsch
Moving Object Detection and Segmentation for Remote Aerial Video Surveillance. 2015
ISBN 978-3-7315-0320-0

Band 19 Marco Huber
Nonlinear Gaussian Filtering: Theory, Algorithms, and Applications. 2015
ISBN 978-3-7315-0338-5

Band 20 Jürgen Beyerer, Alexey Pak (Hrsg.)
Proceedings of the 2014 Joint Workshop of Fraunhofer IOSB and Institute for Anthropomatics, Vision and Fusion Laboratory. 2014
ISBN 978-3-7315-0401-6

Band 21 Todor Dimitrov
Permanente Optimierung dynamischer Probleme der Fertigungssteuerung unter Einbeziehung von Benutzerinteraktionen. 2015
ISBN 978-3-7315-0426-9

Band 22 Benjamin Kühn
Interessengetriebene audiovisuelle Szenenexploration. 2016
ISBN 978-3-7315-0457-3

Band 23 Yvonne Fischer
Wissensbasierte probabilistische Modellierung für die Situationsanalyse am Beispiel der maritimen Überwachung. 2016
ISBN 978-3-7315-0460-3

Band 24 Jürgen Beyerer, Alexey Pak (Hrsg.)
Proceedings of the 2015 Joint Workshop of Fraunhofer IOSB and Institute for Anthropomatics, Vision and Fusion Laboratory. 2016
ISBN 978-3-7315-0519-8